CONSTIPATION – CAUSES, DIAGNOSIS AND TREATMENT

Edited by **Anthony G. Catto-Smith**

Constipation – Causes, Diagnosis and Treatment
Edited by Anthony G. Catto-Smith

Published by InTech

Janeza Trdine 9, 51000 Rijeka, Croatia

Notice

Publishing Process Manager Martina Blecic

Technical Editor Teodora Smiljanic

Cover Designer InTech Design Team

Additional hard copies can be obtained from orders@intechopen.com

Constipation – Causes, Diagnosis and Treatment, Edited by Anthony G. Catto-Smith
p. cm.
ISBN 978-953-51-0237-3

For EU product safety concerns:
IN TECH d.o.o., Prolaz Marije Krucifikse Kozulić 3, 51000 Rijeka, Croatia,
info@intechopen.com or visit our website at intechopen.com.

Meet the editor

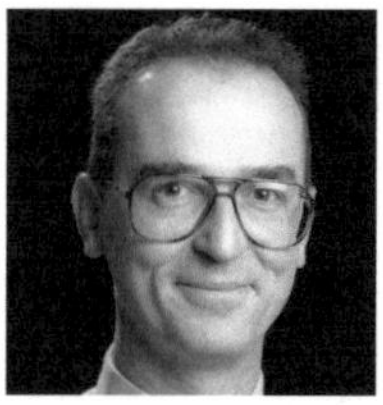

Professor Tony G Catto-Smith is Director of the Department of Gastroenterology and Clinical Nutrition at the Royal Children's Hospital, Melbourne. He qualified in medicine from St Bartholomew's Hospital in London, trained in paediatrics in the UK and Australia, then in paediatric gastroenterology at the University of Calgary in Canada. After returning to Melbourne in 1990, he pioneered the introduction of clinical techniques for the measurement of gastrointestinal motility at RCH. He has continued a strong clinical interest in disorders of colorectal function and published extensively in this area. A major clinical achievement has been the introduction of percutaneous endoscopic gastrostomy placement for children in Australia. Other clinical and research interests include the pathogenesis and treatment of Crohn's and Ulcerative Colitis. He is the author of over 100 journal articles.

Contents

Preface

Constipation is common in both adults and children. Estimates would suggest a median prevalence of around 12-16% in the general population.[1] While regarded as a minor nuisance in some cases, its consequences can be severe, with a substantial impact on quality of life.[2] Secondary faecal soiling has a profound psychological effect at all ages.

This book provides specific contributions which clarify the pathogenesis, diagnosis, and therapy of constipation for the general population and also for certain high risk groups.

Surprisingly, consensus definitions of constipation have been hard to achieve, but that achieved by the PACCT group[3] for children included having at least 2 of the following features within the last 8 weeks:

- Fewer than 3 bowel movements per week
- More than one episode of fecal incontinence per week
- Large stools in the rectum or palpable on abdominal examination
- Passing of stools so large that they obstruct the toilet
- Retentive posturing and withholding behavior
- Painful defecation.

Importantly, it may not be recognised, only coming to attention because of abdominal pain, soiling or behavioural disturbances. The chapter by Kathleen McGrath critically examines the impact defaecation disorders have in children and the diagnostic criteria used to identify them.

Defaecation disorders are also much more prevalent in certain groups. The very young and the elderly[4, 5] are at particular risk. They also pose a particular difficulty for both children and adults with developmental disabilities[6], neurological dysfunction and spinal cord injury.[7] Medical and surgical therapy may also lead to constipation through the use of potent analgesics such as opiods. The chapters by Caterina Aurilio and Kelly Sprawls provide insights into the aetiology of opiod-induced constipation and pharmaceutical approaches to avoiding it and its therapy. Occasionally, constipation may be the presenting feature of another condition such as thyroid disease or colorectal malignancy.[8] The relationship between colorectal tumors and colonoscopy is addressed in the chapter by Brusciano. The chapters by Luca Galleli and Elsie Gulick provide insights into the impact of the broad spectrum of neurological disorders and multiple sclerosis respectively on colorectal dysfunction.

In most situations, constipation occurs in otherwise well individuals. The pathogenesis in these cases is usually proposed to be inadequate dietary fibre, a sedentary lifestyle, or poor toileting techniques. The chapter by Tomoko Fujiwara provides an insightful and unique window into the impact of the all too common habit of skipping breakfast on bowel function.

Diagnosis is usually straightforward, but it often helpful to make reference to diagnostic criteria such as that achieved by the PACCT group. Further diagnostic testing is not usually required, but can be invaluable in specific instances. The chapter on diagnostic tests (Catto-Smith et al.) provides a review of the available testing techniques. While abdominal radiography is often employed, it is rarely adds much. Studies of colorectal motility[9, 10] provide an immense amount of information but are either expensive, invasive, or difficult to interpret[11]. However, they have enabled a better understanding of the motility dysfunction responsible for constipation.[12] Sensory dysfunction is clearly important as many patients are unaware of the extent of rectal filling.[13] These type of studies have however meant that entities such as slow transit constipation, anorectal incoordination, sphincteric dysfunction and the basis for constipation in irritable bowel syndrome are now much better understood[14]. The chapter by Brian Dobson provides a novel hypothesis into the pathogenesis of defaecation disorders in irritable bowel syndrome.

In many situations, otherwise uncomplicated constipation will respond to simple interventions such as attention to diet[15] and toileting, but in other patients it can be extraordinarily difficult to achieve therapeutic success. Medications generally function through either assisting colorectal contractility or softening the stool.[16] Unfortunately, drugs only offer temporary relief if the primary cause is unable to be improved. Recent interest has centred on possibly dysbiotic colonic flora in the hope that probiotics[17] may be helpful. There are a variety of traditional and complementary medications that are used widely in the community.[18]

Behavioural therapies are often very effective in children,[19, 20] and biofeedback modalities have attracted a great deal of interest, particularly in adults. [21]

Better understanding of the pathophysiology of defaecation disorders has opened the doors to novel treatments. Abnormalities in the excitatory cells primarily responsible controlling gastrointestinal motility have been postulated to have a major role in certain types of constipation such as slow transit[22] and even that associated with diabetes.[23] The chapter by Christian Breuer provides a good understanding of the Interstitial Cell of Cajal – a central player in gastrointestinal dysmotility and slow transit constipation. Sacral stimulation is certainly effective, but is invasive. A very exciting new area is that of transabdominal electrical stimulation, [24] which appears to offer the unenviable combination of low cost, ease of use, durability of effect to an otherwise treatment-resistant population.[25, 26]

It goes without saying that the introduction of any new therapy must be accompanied by careful evaluation. The chapter by Scott Harris provides a careful and clear description of the core aspects of clinical development and trials of a range of therapeutic modalities in chronic idiopathic constipation.

Anthony G. Catto-Smith
The Royal Children's Hospital, Melbourne,
Australia

References

[1] Mugie SM, Benninga MA, Di Lorenzo C. Epidemiology of constipation in children and adults: a systematic review. Best Practice & Research in Clinical Gastroenterology 2011;25:3-18.
[2] Wald A, Sigurdsson L. Quality of life in children and adults with constipation. Best Practice & Research in Clinical Gastroenterology 2011;25:19-27.
[3] Benninga M, Candy DC, Catto-Smith AG, Clayden G, Loening-Baucke V, Di Lorenzo C, Nurko S, Staiano A. The Paris Consensus on Childhood Constipation Terminology (PACCT) Group. J Pediatr Gastroenterol Nutr 2005;40:273-5.
[4] McCrea GL, Miaskowski C, Stotts NA, Macera L, Varma MG. A review of the literature on gender and age differences in the prevalence and characteristics of constipation in North America. Journal of Pain & Symptom Management 2009;37:737-45.
[5] Gallagher P, O'Mahony D. Constipation in old age. Best Practice & Research in Clinical Gastroenterology 2009;23:875-87.
[6] Matson JL, LoVullo SV. Encopresis, soiling and constipation in children and adults with developmental disability. Research in Developmental Disabilities 2009;30:799-807.
[7] Lynch AC, Anthony A, Dobbs BR, Frizelle FA. Anorectal physiology following spinal cord injury. Spinal Cord 2000;38:573-80.
[8] Astin M, Griffin T, Neal RD, Rose P, Hamilton W. The diagnostic value of symptoms for colorectal cancer in primary care: a systematic review. British Journal of General Practice 2011;61:e231-43.
[9] Southwell BR, Clarke MC, Sutcliffe J, Hutson JM. Colonic transit studies: normal values for adults and children with comparison of radiological and scintigraphic methods. Pediatric Surgery International 2009;25:559-72.
[10] Dinning PG, Benninga MA, Southwell BR, Scott SM. Paediatric and adult colonic manometry: a tool to help unravel the pathophysiology of constipation. World Journal of Gastroenterology 2010;16:5162-72.
[11] Quigley EM. What we have learned about colonic motility: normal and disturbed. Current Opinion in Gastroenterology 2010;26:53-60.

[12] King SK, Catto-Smith AG, Stanton MP, Sutcliffe JR, Simpson D, Cook I, Dinning P, Hutson JM, Southwell BR. 24-Hour colonic manometry in pediatric slow transit constipation shows significant reductions in antegrade propagation. American Journal of Gastroenterology 2008;103:2083-91.

[13] Scott SM, van den Berg MM, Benninga MA. Rectal sensorimotor dysfunction in constipation. Best Practice & Research in Clinical Gastroenterology 2011;25:103-18.

[14] Dinning PG, Di Lorenzo C. Colonic dysmotility in constipation. Best Practice & Research in Clinical Gastroenterology 2011;25:89-101.

[15] Suares NC, Ford AC. Systematic review: the effects of fibre in the management of chronic idiopathic constipation. Alimentary Pharmacology & Therapeutics 2011;33:895-901.

[16] Ford AC, Suares NC. Effect of laxatives and pharmacological therapies in chronic idiopathic constipation: systematic review and meta-analysis. Gut 2011;60:209-18.

[17] Chmielewska A, Szajewska H. Systematic review of randomised controlled trials: probiotics for functional constipation. World Journal of Gastroenterology 2010;16:69-75.

[18] Cheng CW, Bian ZX, Wu TX. Systematic review of Chinese herbal medicine for functional constipation. World Journal of Gastroenterology 2009;15:4886-95.

[19] Catto-Smith AG. 5. Constipation and toileting issues in children. Med J Aust 2005;182:242-6.

[20] Whitehead WE, di Lorenzo C, Leroi AM, Porrett T, Rao SS. Conservative and behavioural management of constipation. Neurogastroenterology & Motility 2009;21 Suppl 2:55-61.

[21] Koh CE, Young CJ, Young JM, Solomon MJ. Systematic review of randomized controlled trials of the effectiveness of biofeedback for pelvic floor dysfunction. British Journal of Surgery 2008;95:1079-87.

[22] Sutcliffe J, King SK, Clarke MC, Farmer P, Hutson JM, Southwell BR. Reduced distribution of pacemaking cells in dilated colon. Pediatric Surgery International 2007;23:1179-82.

[23] Southwell BR, Southwell BR. Loss of interstitial cells of Cajal may be central to poor intestinal motility in diabetes mellitus. Journal of Gastroenterology & Hepatology 2008;23:505-7.

[24] van Wunnik BP, Baeten CG, Southwell BR. Neuromodulation for constipation: sacral and transcutaneous stimulation. Best Practice & Research in Clinical Gastroenterology 2011;25:181-91.

[25] Ismail KA, Chase J, Gibb S, Clarke M, Catto-Smith AG, Robertson VJ, Hutson JM, Southwell BR. Daily transabdominal electrical stimulation at home increased defecation in children with slow-transit constipation: a pilot study. Journal of Pediatric Surgery 2009;44:2388-92.

[26] Clarke MC, Chase JW, Gibb S, Robertson VJ, Catto-Smith A, Hutson JM, Southwell BR. Decreased colonic transit time after transcutaneous interferential electrical stimulation in children with slow transit constipation. Journal of Pediatric Surgery 2009;44:408-12.

1

Diagnostic Approach to Constipation in Children

Kathleen H. McGrath[1] and Patrina Caldwell[2]
[1]*The Royal Children's Hospital, Melbourne*
[2]*University of Sydney, The Children's Hospital at Westmead, Sydney*
Australia

1. Introduction

Constipation is a common paediatric problem. It is relevant to the practice of both general paediatricians and paediatric gastroenterologists and accounts for 3% and 25% of outpatient visits respectively (Levine, 1975; Taitz et al., 1986). International prevalence rates range from 0.7% to 29.6% which is similar for males and females (van den Berg et al., 2006). The broad range of reported prevalence is related to differing criteria for defining constipation but may also reflect genuine differences between ethnic populations and socioeconomic influences.

The diagnosis of constipation is historically a subjective and symptom-based approach. It relies on good clinical history taking and physical examination, in particular to exclude an underlying organic aetiology. In order to objectify the classification of this entity and allow for comparison of data between studies (e.g. prevalence rates, treatment outcomes), a number of diagnostic classifications have been proposed. This chapter will discuss the origin of these various classifications, their application and role within paediatric clinical practice and research. It will also provide a suggested clinical approach to the diagnosis of constipation in children, including the problems that may be encountered.

2. Importance of the appropriate diagnosis of constipation in children

Symptoms of childhood constipation may vary from mild and short-lived to severe and chronic. It can affect children in all age groups from infants to adolescents and can extend into adulthood.

Constipation is associated with a wide range of consequences for the individual child. These include physical pain and discomfort, psychological distress (primarily related to faecal incontinence) and an increased risk of urinary dysfunction. It can also impact on quality of life, family dynamics and socialisation through missed days of school and work (Belsey et al., 2010). In some children, a delayed or missed diagnosis can result in progression towards a significant chronic health problem with physical, psychological and social implications.

2.1 Impact on the child: Physical discomfort associated with constipation

Constipation is associated with varying degrees of physical discomfort for children. The onset of constipation is often related to experience(s) of painful defaecation. This may be caused by the presence of an anal fissure, perianal infection or perianal inflammation due to cow's milk protein intolerance or other underlying medical conditions. Once children experience discomfort, they commonly associate the process of defaecation with pain and actively attempt to avoid it. This may manifest as toilet refusal or stool withholding behaviours where there is voluntary contraction of the external anal sphincter with the urge to defaecate.

Repetitive withholding behaviours result in further constipation as the brain begins to ignore the signals that would usually alert the child to the need to defaecate (Weaver & Dobson, 2007). This results in stools that are hard, large and difficult to pass which can lead to further experiences of pain and the development of perianal tears, perpetuating the cycle of painful defaecation, stool withholding and worsening constipation.

Constipation is one of the most frequent causes for abdominal pain in children presenting to their medical practitioner or the emergency department. One study found that acute or chronic constipation accounted for 48% of children with acute abdominal pain presenting to a large academic paediatric primary care population (Loening-Baucke & Swidsinski, 2007).

Ongoing chronic constipation results in stool impaction, distension of the rectum and sigmoid colon and rectal insensitivity. Stool impaction can cause abdominal pain which may vary from mild to severe in nature. Children with constipation may also experience systemic symptoms including loss of appetite, nausea, vomiting and weight loss.

2.2 Impact on the child: Chronic constipation and quality of life

Constipation can affect a child's physical and mental wellbeing and impact on their overall quality of life. Section 2.1 described the common physical manifestations of constipation including pain.

Studies have further assessed the impact of chronic constipation on a child's emotional status. One Australian study assessed a cohort of children with slow transit constipation (confirmed on radioisotope study) and compared them with a group of healthy children with normal bowel patterns. The study found that children with constipation reported a significantly lower quality of life (assessed by questionnaires addressing domains of physical, emotional, social and school functioning) compared with the non-constipated children. In addition, the parents of these children reported a significantly lower quality of life for their child than the child's self-reporting using the same scoring system (Clarke et al, 2008). Constipation not only affects the individual child's quality of life, but may impact on their relationship with parents and / or siblings and the family dynamics as a whole.

Another study compared children with constipation to groups of children with inflammatory bowel disease, gastro-oesophageal reflux disease or normal health. They found that children with constipation reported a significantly lower quality of life (assessed by self and parental reporting) compared with both healthy children and children with inflammatory bowel disease or gastro-oesophageal reflux disease (Youssef et al., 2005). This was a pertinent finding considering that inflammatory bowel disease is traditionally accepted by physicians and the general population as being a more serious condition than constipation.

A recent systematic review by Belsey and colleagues demonstrated that impaired quality of life is a consistent finding in children and adults with chronic constipation. They found that the quality of life in children with chronic constipation was comparable to those of children with other chronic conditions traditionally regarded as being more serious, including cardiac and rheumatologic diseases (Belsey et al., 2010).

The diagnosis of chronic constipation in children should be taken seriously as its impact on quality of life may be far greater than initially anticipated. It should be considered a public health issue for primary physicians, paediatricians and paediatric gastroenterologists. Further studies are needed to specifically assess the impact of this condition on quality of life when it lasts from childhood into adulthood.

2.3 Impact on the child: Faecal incontinence and psychological distress

Faecal incontinence refers to the passage of stools in an inappropriate place (Benninga et al., 2005). It occurs in 1-3% of children and can affect up to 8% of adults (Catto-Smith, 2005). Faecal incontinence is a frequent accompanying symptom of childhood constipation. Studies show that it is present in up to 84% of children with constipation (Vooskijl et al., 2004). In around 80% of cases of faecal incontinence, it is involuntary and occurs in the setting of chronic constipation (constipation-associated faecal incontinence) (Joinson et al., 2006). Less commonly faecal incontinence can be voluntary (non-retentive faecal incontinence) and may be related to emotional disturbance with no evidence of constipation being present.

Functional constipation and stool withholding behaviours lead to impaction of faeces in the rectum, distension of the rectum and sigmoid colon and rectal insensitivity which may result in faecal incontinence. Due to rectal insensitivity, children may not be aware of this happening. Risk factors for faecal incontinence are listed in Table 1.

Faecal incontinence is associated with behavioural and emotional problems in children. A recent population study of over 8000 children found significantly higher rates of behavioural and emotional problems in children with faecal incontinence compared to those without. In addition they noted that these problems were significantly greater in children who soiled frequently compared with those who soiled only occasionally (less than once per week) (Joinson et al., 2006).

Children may be embarrassed by their faecal incontinence, associated body odour and differences from their peers. This is particularly the case for school-aged children who may

Risk factor	Other related factors
Chronic constipation	Low dietary fibre and fluid intake Cow's milk protein intolerance Poor toilet posture and incomplete evacuation Medical conditions (hypothyroidism, hypercalcaemia, hypokalaemia) Medications
Toilet refusal	Previous painful defaecation Commencement of school
Psychological factors	Autistic spectrum disorders Attention deficit hyperactivity disorder Significant emotional life events

Table 1. Risk factors for faecal incontinence (modified from Ho & Caldwell, 2008).

experience teasing or bullying and social isolation. Constant focus on the child's bowel habits from the parents may distress the child and cause conflict within the home between family members. Parents may wrongly 'blame' the child for being 'lazy' and punish them unnecessarily, causing further emotional distress. The child's degree of distress and low self-esteem may affect their behaviour and cause them to become withdrawn or alternatively 'act up'. There may be considerable negative implications on their learning and performance at school. Further consequences may include missed days of school and work for parents, leading to societal costs on a wider scale.

2.4 Impact on the child: Urinary dysfunction

Epidemiological studies have identified an association between constipation and certain urological conditions. These include urinary incontinence, vesicoureteric reflux and urinary tract infections (McGrath & Caldwell, 2008; Loening-Baucke, 1997; O'Regan et al., 1985, 1986). Loening-Baucke assessed 234 children with chronic constipation and found that 29% had daytime urinary incontinence and 11% had a urinary tract infection. A more recent Australian study found a prevalence of constipation of 36.1% in a population of children with nocturnal enuresis (McGrath & Caldwell, 2008), which is higher than reported international prevalence rates of 0.7% to 29.6% in the normal population.

With successful treatment of constipation, many of these urinary symptoms will resolve. In one study, successful treatment of constipation after 12 months resulted in resolution of daytime urinary incontinence in 89% and urinary tract infection in all patients with normal urinary tract anatomy (Loening-Baucke, 1997).

2.5 Impact on the child: Outcome of late or missed diagnosis

A timely diagnosis of constipation can help to prevent or minimise many of the complications outlined above. If constipation is identified early, management can be initiated in the form of education, toileting programs, dietary modification, behavioural therapy and laxatives. Successful intervention to 'keep the rectum empty' will avoid progression to stool impaction, rectal distension and insensitivity and the onset of faecal incontinence. In addition, the early identification and management of constipation has been shown to result in better treatment response and outcomes (Van Ginkel et al., 2003). This was particularly the case when children were referred for management of constipation under the age of 2 years (Loening-Baucke, 1993).

Missed or delayed diagnosis of constipation can increase the risk of both physical and psychological complications, making the problem more difficult to manage later on. Where urinary dysfunction exists in the context of chronic constipation, a missed diagnosis of constipation may result in treatment failure. An accurate diagnosis of constipation is paramount for provision of optimal patient care and quality of life.

3. The use of diagnostic criteria in childhood constipation

3.1 Definitions and Historical overview

The term 'constipation' derives from the Latin 'constipare' meaning to crowd together. The accepted understanding of constipation describes a constellation of different symptoms related to difficult passage of stool. These may include infrequent passage of stool, firm stool consistency, straining and painful defaecation, retentive posturing and faecal incontinence. The subjective nature of these symptoms has historically made defining and diagnosing constipation a challenge and there is no consensus on the definition for 'constipation'. This has limited the ability of researchers to accurately compare different clinical studies in this field and accounts in part for the wide range of reported international prevalence.

In an attempt to standardise the definition of constipation and the related disorders of gastrointestinal motility, diagnostic criteria were created. Generally, these separate functional constipation from that secondary to medical illnesses and medications. They are outlined below and summarised in Table 2.

Early attempts to formalise a definition of constipation included the Iowa classic criteria. This classification was used by some groups in clinical research for the last two decades but its application in clinical practice was sporadic and the mainstream diagnosis of constipation remained largely subjective.

In 1989, a group of investigators met in Rome to form a consensus opinion to assist in the diagnosis of functional gastrointestinal disorders (FGID). Initially the group focussed on the adult population. In 1997, at a consensus conference, the Rome I Criteria were discussed with relation to childhood, forming the Paediatric Rome II Criteria (published in 1999). Also in 1997, the Bristol Stool Chart was published as an aid for classification of stool by appearance and consistency (Lewis & Heaton, 1997) (see Figure 1). Interpretation of these illustrations was extrapolated to help assist in the diagnosis of constipation (Table 2).

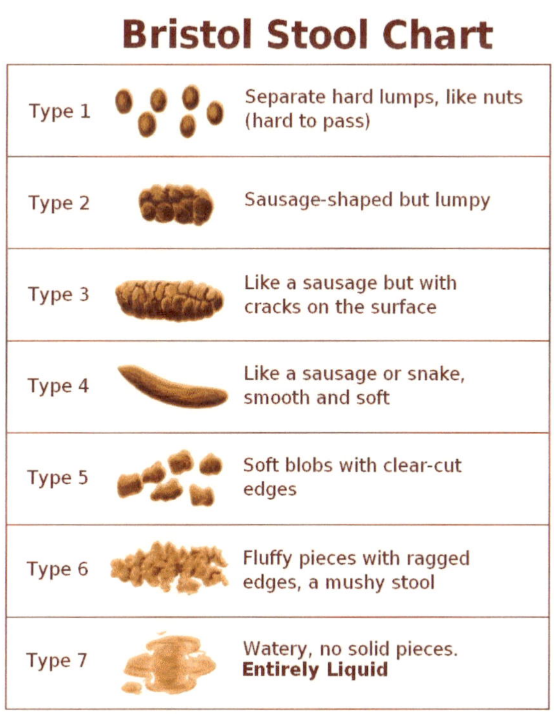

Fig. 1. Bristol stool chart (Lewis and Heaton, 1997).

Bristol stool chart (see Fig. 1.)
Constipation indicated by Types 1 and 2
(Types 4 > 3 being the 'ideal stools' and Types 5 to 7 tending towards diarrhoea)
(Lewis & Heaton, 1997)

Classic Iowa criteria
Paediatric constipation = at least 2 of the following criteria:

- Defecation frequency <3 times per week
- Two or more encopresis episodes per week
- Periodic passage of very large amounts of stool once every 7 to 30 days (the criterion of a large amount of stool is satisfied if it is estimated to be twice the standard amount of stool, shown in a clay model, or is stools are so large that they clog the toilet).

Solitary encopresis = in a child older than 4 years of age:

- Two or more encopresis episodes per week
- Defecation frequency ≥3 times per week

No passage of very large amounts of stool
(Loening-Baucke, 1990, as cited in Benninga et al., 2004)

Rome II criteria
Functional constipation: In infants and preschool children (from 1 month to 6 years), at least 2 weeks of

- Scybalous, pebble-like, hard stools in a majority of stools, or
- Firm stools 2 or fewer times/week, and
- No evidence of structural, endocrine, or metabolic disease

Functional faecal retention: From infancy to 16 years old, a history of at least 12 weeks of

- Passage of large-diameter stools at intervals <2 times/week, and
- Retentive posturing, avoiding defecation by purposefully contracting the pelvic floor. As pelvic floor muscles fatigue, the child uses the gluteal muscles, squeezing the buttocks together.

Functional non-retentive faecal soiling: Once a week or more for the preceding 12 weeks, in a child over age 4 years, a history of defaecation

- In places and at times inappropriate to the social context
- In the absence of structural or inflammatory disease, and

In the absence of signs of faecal retention.
(Rasquin-Weber et al., 1999)

Working group report of the first world congress of Paediatric Gastroenterology, Hepatology, and Nutrition
Constipation is a symptom defined by the occurrence of any of the following, independent of stool frequency:

- Passage of hard, scybalous, pebble-like or cylindrical cracked stools
- Straining or painful defecation

- Passage of large stools that may clog the toilet

Or stool frequency less than 3 per week, unless the child is breast fed.
(Hyams et al., 2002)

PACCT criteria
Chronic constipation: Occurrence of 2 or more of the following characteristics during the preceding 8 weeks:

- Fewer than 3 bowel movements per week
- More than 1 episode of faecal incontinence/week
- Large stools in the rectum or palpable on abdominal examination
- Passage of large-diameter stools that may obstruct the toilet
- Display of retentive posturing and withholding behaviours
- Painful defecation

Faecal incontinence: Passage of stools in an inappropriate place

- *Organic faecal incontinence*: faecal incontinence resulting from organic disease
- *Functional faecal incontinence*: nonorganic disease that can be subdivided into:
  - Constipation-associated faecal incontinence: functional faecal incontinence associated with the presence of constipation
  - Non-retentive (non-constipation-associated) faecal incontinence: passage of stools in an inappropriate place, occurring in children with a mental age of 4 years and older, with no evidence of constipation based on history and/or examination

(Benninga et al., 2005)

Rome III criteria
Functional constipation: Must include <u>1 month</u> of at least 2 of the following in <u>infants up to 4 years of age:</u>

- Two or fewer defecations per week
- At least 1 episode per week of incontinence after the acquisition of toileting skills
- History of excessive stool retention
- History of painful or hard bowel movements
- Presence of a large faecal mass in the rectum
- History of large-diameter stools that may obstruct the toilet

(Hyman et al., 2006)

Functional constipation: Must include 2 or more of the following in a child with a developmental age of <u>at least 4 years</u> with insufficient criteria for diagnosis of irritable bowel syndrome:

- Two or fewer defecations in the toilet per week
- At least 1 episode of faecal incontinence per week
- History of retentive posturing or excessive volitional stool retention
- History of painful or hard bowel movements
- Presence of a large faecal mass in the rectum
- History of large-diameter stools that may obstruct the toilet

Criteria must be fulfilled at least once per week for <u>at least 2 months</u> before diagnosis
(Rasquin et al., 2006)

Non-retentive faecal incontinence: Must include all of the following in a child with a developmental age of at least 4 years: • Defecation into places inappropriate to the social context at least once per month • No evidence of an inflammatory, anatomic, metabolic or neoplastic process that • explains the subject's symptoms No evidence of faecal retention.

Table 2. Different classification for childhood constipation.

Some paediatric gastroenterologists and paediatricians found the symptom based Paediatric Rome II Criteria to be too restrictive (see section 3.2). In light of this, a group of experts (paediatric gastroenterologists and paediatricians) gathered in Paris in 2004 to redefine working definitions in gastrointestinal motility (The Paris Consensus on Childhood Constipation Terminology (PACCT) Group). The definition of functional constipation described by PACCT was published in its own right in 2005.

PACCT also recommended discontinuation of the terms 'encopresis' and 'soiling' and replacement by the term 'faecal incontinence'. Soiling was a term that had often been used mutually with encopresis but was felt by the PACCT group to be too broad with possible negative connotations of dirtiness and blame in some cultures. Likewise, the term encopresis was used widely with variable degrees of interpretation and understanding. Some clinicians used this term to refer to intentional passage of stool in a socially inappropriate place (often associated with a psychological disorder). It was thought that discontinuing these two terms in favour of the more strictly defined 'faecal incontinence' would lead to more agreement in understanding and a greater capacity to properly compare different clinical studies. Faecal incontinence was defined as passage of stools in an inappropriate place. For the purposes of this chapter, we will use the term 'faecal incontinence' in place of 'encopresis' or 'soiling', including where studies were published prior to PACCT in 2005.

PACCT was further used to assist in the development of the Rome III Criteria (published in 2006). The Rome III Criteria addressed previously perceived problems such as age restriction (infants versus children / adolescents) and retentive posturing as a component symptom which will be discussed in more detail in Section 3.2.

3.2 Comparison and contrast of diagnostic classifications for constipation

There continues to be varying opinions on the benefits and limitations of the different diagnostic classifications for constipation. The intention behind their derivation was to 'objectify' the ability to diagnose constipation, to allow for comparison between clinical research studies and to aid in the identification of this common paediatric problem in clinical practice. Table 3 summarises the various differences and similarities between the criteria of the classification systems. Below, we have provided a more detailed description of the comparison and contrast between these classifications.

In order to be useful, a diagnostic classification must be shown to be reliable, valid and applicable for a range of relevant population groups. There were a few early attempts to validate the Rome II criteria for functional gastrointestinal disorders. Some studies found the Rome II criteria were helpful for diagnosing functional gastrointestinal disorders in childhood however these studies were conducted in a tertiary setting, and may not be generalisable (Miele et al., 2004; Caplan et al., 2005).

Classification	Frequency of stools	Faecal incontinence	Large stool size-rectal or abdominal exam	Large stool size-toilet	Stool withholding / Retention	Painful Defaecation	Stool Consistency
Iowa criteria	√	√	-	√	-	-	-
Rome II	√	-	-	-	-	-	√
Working group	√	-	-	√	-	√	√
PACCT	√	√	√	√	√	√	-
Rome III	√	√	√	√	√	√	√

Table 3. Comparison of criteria of different classifications for childhood constipation

Since their origin, the Rome II criteria have been widely criticised for being too restrictive. Studies have compared the diagnosis of constipation by the Rome II criteria with other classification systems. One study compared the Rome II criteria with the classic Iowa criteria in identification of constipation in 198 otherwise healthy children referred to a tertiary centre for defaecation disorders. They found the prevalence of constipation was 69% by the Rome II criteria and 74% by the classic Iowa criteria (Voskijl et al., 2004). These results suggest that some children may be missed by the Rome II criteria. A similar study from Turkey assessing children referred to general paediatric or paediatric gastroenterology units for constipation found a prevalence of 72.5% by the Iowa criteria compared with 63.7% by the Rome II criteria (Aydogdu et al., 2009).

One of the main aspects of the Rome II criteria which has restricted its capacity for identification of constipation in children is its exclusion of faecal incontinence as a criterion. Faecal incontinence is common and may affect up to 84% of constipated children (Vooskijl et al., 2004). Exclusion of this relatively frequent symptom may lead to under diagnosis. This was illustrated in the study by Voskijl et al comparing the Rome II diagnostic criteria with the classic Iowa criteria. 16% of children diagnosed with constipation by the classic Iowa criteria did not fulfil the Rome II criteria. These children had low defaecation frequency in combination with encopresis and / or faecal retention (Voskijl et al., 2004). Faecal incontinence is not part of the Rome II criteria. This was considered in creation of the PACCT and Rome III criteria in 2004 and 2006 respectively, with inclusion of 'faecal incontinence more than once per week' as a component criterion for these classifications.

Another group assessed the prevalence of functional defaecation disorders (including constipation) according to PACCT versus Rome II criteria and attempted to compare their clinical validity (Boccia et al., 2007). They found that 53 of 126 (42.1%) of children defined as constipated by PACCT criteria were not recognised by the Rome II criteria, and one child was diagnosed as constipated by Rome II criteria and not PACCT. Many of the children missed by Rome II criteria were excluded purely on the basis of its age restrictions (i.e. not between 1 month and 6 years). This criterion excludes all children greater than 6 years old with constipation regardless of whether they fulfil the other symptom criteria. This stringency is likely to fail to diagnose constipation in older children and supports previous opinion that the Rome II criteria are too restrictive.

In 2005, the PACCT criteria attempted to provide an expert consensus on working definitions in childhood defaecation disorders. The two most pertinent changes were the unification of 'Rome II functional constipation' and 'functional faecal retention' to 'chronic constipation' and the replacement of the terms 'soiling' and 'encopresis' with 'faecal incontinence'. Stool withholding behaviours or retentive posturing was also included as a new criterion although some physicians feel these behaviours may be difficult for parents to recognise in their child.

The Rome III criteria are really an extension of the PACCT criteria but with different duration requirements for different age groups (symptoms for at least 1 month in infants/ children under 4 years old and for at least 2 months in children older than 4 years). With regard to symptom duration, the reduced requirement from symptoms of 3 months duration to 1 month (in infants / toddlers) and to 2 months in children greater than 4 years old/ adolescents was one of the pertinent changes from Rome II to Rome III. This was particularly important in light of recognition that earlier identification of constipation and treatment intervention is associated with a better treatment response and outcome.

There are some studies comparing the Rome III and PACCT classifications. Many of these studies were conducted in populations of children referred to tertiary centres and so their results may not be generalisable to children in the community. One study from Sri Lanka which may be more applicable to children in the community compared Rome III and PACCT criteria for diagnosing constipation among school children aged 10-16 years old. They performed a cross-sectional survey in 5 classes randomly selected from a semi-urban school using a validated, self administered questionnaire with guidance from research assistants. The prevalence of constipation was 10.7% by both the Rome III and PACCT criteria suggesting a level of agreement between the classifications (Rajindrajith et al., 2009).

One criticism of PACCT has been the exclusion of 'scybalous, pebble-like stools' as a criterion for constipation. Some groups have shown that a high percentage of constipated children report this symptom and advocate for its inclusion in future diagnostic criteria (Boccia et al., 2007; Maffei & Morais, 2005). The Rome III classification does not directly refer to this condition but does have 'history of painful or hard bowel movements' as one of its criteria which may incorporate this criterion. Similarly, straining that is not accompanied by pain has been suggested for inclusion in future classifications in light of its relatively frequent reporting in constipated children. One recent study in Sri Lanka identified straining in 75% of children with constipation (as defined by both the PACCT and Rome III criteria) (Rajindrajith et al., 2009).

Another criticism of PACCT has been that 'large faecal mass in the rectum' (a criteria only ascertained by physical examination or an abdominal radiograph) may be difficult to assess in large community surveys (without the involvement of an assessing clinician) (Maffei and Morais, 2005). There is a strong need to address the applicability and validity of the Rome III diagnostic classification for constipation in both primary care and community settings.

Some of the above concerns were addressed by the 'Boston working group' in their definition of constipation in children (Hyams et al, 2002) (see Table 2). This is another diagnostic classification which takes into account that not all constipated children may have infrequent defaecation. It also accounts for the known variation in stool consistency amongst breastfed infants and wide variant of the norm.

The evolution of these diagnostic classifications reflects the complexities of trying to create a system that can be easily understood, reliable, applicable to children in both hospital and community settings and validated by evidence based processes.

4. Challenges associated with the diagnosis of constipation in the paediatric population

The traditional diagnostic approach centres on a thorough history, detailed examination and the use of relevant supporting investigations. This can be challenging in paediatrics requiring utilisation of the 'art' of medicine to take a history from both child and parents, and willingness to modify the examination of the child depending on age and cooperation.

As current definitions of constipation are largely symptom based, the reporting of these symptoms is influenced by an individual's perception of 'the norm'. Studies have shown that parents and children may have different insight into a child's symptoms (Caplan et al., 2005), which may pose a further challenge for clinicians.

4.1 Different insight from parents, clinicians and children

Constipation can be difficult for parents to recognise and they may under-report this condition in their child. There is a difference between parental and clinician recognition of constipation.

One study found that parents tended to under-report constipation in their children (sensitivity 23%) but were good at recognising when their child was not constipated (specificity 90%) (McGrath & Caldwell, 2008). Although parents were able to identify individual symptoms of constipation during history taking, they were poor at recognising that these symptoms signified constipation. Table 4 outlines the recognition of different symptoms of constipation by parents in this cohort. Parents were more likely to report constipation with infrequent defecation and presence of faecal incontinence. There was no significant association between parental reporting of constipation and hard consistency of stools and the presence of straining during defaecation.

Clinicians should carefully question parents and children about individual symptoms of constipation rather than relying on parents to recognise that their child is constipated. Other influential factors that must be addressed in history-taking include whether the child is toilet trained, the ease of toilet training, how 'involved' the parents are in their child's bowel hygiene (i.e. do they still require assistance after defaecation with wiping / redressing) and whether the reporting parent is the primary carer for the child (how much time do they spend attending to the child's daily needs). The use of a stool diary may be of value in improving the reliability of recall of this information.

Despite carefully worded questions during history taking, symptoms of constipation may still be missed secondary to parental misunderstanding. Faecal incontinence may be mistaken by parents as 'poor wiping technique by the child' rather than as a manifestation of underlying constipation. In addition, obstipation (severe persistent constipation) with overflow may present with the passage of soft stools which can be mistaken as diarrhoea or even normal bowel actions.

Parental under-reporting or misunderstanding of symptoms may affect the diagnosis of constipation. Recognition of this common condition may also be affected by unreliable history being given by the child. One study compared reporting of duration of symptoms by child versus parent (supported by dates of medical record documentation or relevant investigations). Children tended to under-report symptom duration (with reports of less than 12 weeks compared with duration of greater than 12 weeks according to parental reporting and documentation). This study also showed a significant disparity between parental and child estimates regarding the frequency of the child's stool symptoms (Schurman et al., 2005). Another study supported similar findings with a low concordance identified between the diagnoses of functional constipation made by parents versus children (Caplan et al., 2005).

Parameters of bowel function as assessed by clinician	Parental reporting of constipation N (%)	Parental reporting of no constipation N (%)	χ^2 p value
Soiling (in last 6 months)			
No	14 (35.9)	130 (56.5)	0.02*
Yes	25 (64.1)	100 (43.5)	
Frequency of defecation			
≥ Daily	16 (41)	140 (60.6)	
A few times per week	21 (53.8)	88 (38.1)	0.03*
< Weekly	2 (5.1)	3 (1.3)	
Straining			
No	13 (33.3)	99 (42.9)	0.3
Yes	26 (66.7)	132 (57.1)	
Consistency of stools			
Soft	2 (5.1)	9 (3.9)	
Normal	25 (64.1)	171 (74.3)	0.4
Hard	12 (30.8)	50 (21.7)	

* Statistically significant result (P<0.05)

Table 4. Parental reporting of constipation compared with individual parameters of bowel function assessed by clinician (used with permission from McGrath & Caldwell, 2008).

These studies and discrepancies between parent and child reporting highlight certain issues specific to the paediatric consultation. At the various ages and stages of childhood development, who (parent or child) is the most appropriate history-giver? There is no easy answer to this but there needs to be a balance of input from the parent and child, and children's opinions should always be sought in the process of the consultation.

4.2 Treating physicians not familiar with diagnostic criteria

Despite the common nature of constipation in paediatric practice, recent evidence suggests that there is a degree of variability in the diagnosis of constipation between clinicians at different levels of health care. At a tertiary level, one study demonstrated low inter-rater reliability for diagnosis of constipation by different Paediatric Gastroenterologists (Saps & Di Lorenzo, 2004).

Because of the limitations in defining constipation, it is difficult to ascertain the true prevalence of this problem in different primary health care settings. However, it is a common problem in the primary care setting and the family doctor is often the one who initiates preliminary diagnosis and management. This is particularly the case in settings where a primary carer referral is required prior to seeing a paediatrician or paediatric specialist. Unfortunately some primary care physicians are not aware of current diagnostic classifications and clinical guidelines for managing constipation in children. One study in the USA found that the majority of primary care physicians (67-86%) in West Virginia were not familiar with the published clinical guidelines for constipation in children (Whitlock-Morales et al., 2007).

Further research is needed to assess the understanding of constipation and its management by primary care physicians and the burden of this condition on their clinical practice. Appropriate clinical updates and education should be provided to primary care physicians as early diagnosis and management is associated with better treatment outcomes.

5. Suggestions for clinical practice: general approach to the diagnosis of constipation in children

5.1 Clinical history-taking

A thorough medical history (taken from the parent and child) is paramount in the diagnosis of constipation in children. It helps to identify the problem, quantify its severity and any complications present and recognise any 'red flags' suggestive of an underlying organic condition (see Table 5).

Parents should be asked about passage of meconium in the newborn period as a delay may indicate underlying Hirschsprung's disease, anorectal malformations including imperforate anus or cystic fibrosis. If cystic fibrosis is suspected, one should clarify whether newborn screening testing has taken place and if not, arrange for appropriate investigations to take place. Details should be sought about the onset of the problem including any associated changes in health status, diet or medications at that particular time.

Certain childhood milestones can be associated with the temporal onset of constipation. These include changes in feeding patterns (e.g. wean from breast milk to cow's milk-based formula or to solid foods) and time of toilet training and details of these milestones should be requested. Enquires should be made about any association between the onset of constipation and the commencement of school. Children may 'put off' defecation when they first start school in order to prioritise play or because they find the school toilet environment unfamiliar or unpleasant. These children may exhibit withholding behaviours or retentive posturing (squeezing legs or buttocks together or often appearing 'fidgety').

Information should be sought about previous treatment strategies used including response to treatment. Questions should be asked directly about stool frequency, consistency (with utilisation of the Bristol Stool Chart as a visual aid), size (e.g. whether they obstruct the toilet bowel), shape (are the stools scybalous or pebble-like), straining during bowel movements (both painful and non-painful), feeling of incomplete bowel emptying or any retentive posturing. Details of associated anorectal pain and episodes of rectal bleeding, mucous in stool or faecal incontinence should be sought. In addition, systemic symptoms should be addressed including abdominal pain, anorexia, fever, nausea, vomiting and weight loss.

Infants and toddlers	**Adolescents**
Unknown	Unknown
Structural problems:	Slow transit constipation
• Anal fissures	Metabolic, systemic problems:
• Anorectal malformations	• Diabetes mellitus
Dietary, behavioural problems:	• Hypothyroidism
• Breast feeding to bottle feeding	• Hypercalcaemia
• Stool withholding behaviour	Toxicity
• Cow's milk protein allergy	• Drugs (opiates, antidepressants, anticholinergics)
Metabolic, systemic problems:	• Lead poisoning
• Coeliac disease	Neoplasia
• Cystic fibrosis	Sexual abuse
Neuroenteric problems:	Psychological problems:
• Intestinal pseudo-obstruction	• Anorexia nervosa
• Hirschsprung's disease	• Depression
• Neuronal intestinal dysplasia	
Spinal cord problems / spina bifida	

Table 5. Organic aetiology of constipation (modified from Benninga et al., 2004).

A dietary and activity history should be determined including fluid intake. Questions should be asked about details of the social environment and any life events of note (e.g. birth of a new sibling, parental separation or family death). Suspected misunderstandings or cultural beliefs related to bowel habits should be explored (such as the belief that faecal incontinence with constipation is from poor wiping technique or voluntary). A history of toileting routines should be sought including whether the child uses a potty or an adult toilet and whether foot support is used.

A strong family history of constipation may be of relevance and the presence of any relatives with possible related conditions such as hypothyroidism or coeliac disease should be clarified. It is important to carefully ask about social circumstances and family dynamics. In particular, one should always ensure there are no concerns about child abuse. It is necessary to exclude any underlying organic aetiology by asking about abdominal distension, ano-sacral malformations, scoliosis, lower limb deformities or neuromuscular signs. In light of its association, urinary dysfunction should be addressed. Details should be asked about daytime and night time incontinence, dysuria, urinary frequency or offensive smelling urine.

5.2 Physical examination

A complete physical and neurologic examination is necessary, focussing on the abdomen, the sacral region (assessing for signs of underlying spinal abnormalities such as skin discolouration, naevi, sinuses, hairy patch or central pit) and the perineum (for the presence of anal fissures and to exclude anal malformations). Anal fissures are commonly associated with painful defaecation and may lead to stool withholding behaviours, chronic constipation, stool impaction and eventually faecal incontinence.

The rectal digital examination is no longer performed as a routine part of examination although some clinicians still employ its use. The clinical benefit of performing this procedure (to assess anal sphincter tone and confirm faecal impaction) must be weighed against the physical and psychological discomfort for the child.

5.3 Role of Investigations

A careful history and detailed examination is all that is required for the diagnosis of most children with functional constipation. In certain situations, there may be a role for investigations including abdominal radiography, blood tests for thyroid disease, coeliac disease or hypercalcaemia, anorectal manometry and colonic transit studies; however this is not discussed further in this chapter.

6. Conclusion

Constipation is a common childhood problem. It affects children of all ages and is relevant to both primary and tertiary care settings. Early identification and treatment of constipation in children is paramount. It has been associated with better response to treatment and overall outcome. Children will experience less associated complications including physical discomfort, impaired quality of life, faecal incontinence and urinary dysfunction.

A number of different symptom based classifications have been created in an attempt to objectify the diagnosis of constipation and allow for better comparison between studies. These classifications have been compared and contrasted but further studies are needed in order to validate their use and encourage widespread acceptance and application.

The diagnosis of constipation in children can be challenging. Parents, children and clinicians may have different opinions on symptoms and may misdiagnose or under-diagnose this condition. Recognition can be optimised by the use of a thorough history and detailed physical examination. In most children, investigations are not required for diagnosis but they may be indicated in some cases of chronic constipation or constipation that is refractory to treatment.

7. References

Aydogdu, S., Cakir, M., Yuksekkaya, H., Arikan, C., Tumgor, G., Baran, M., & Yagci, R. (2009). Chronic constipation in Turkish children: clinical findings and applicability of classification criteria. *The Turkish Journal of Pediatrics*, Vol. 51, pp. 146-153.

Belsey, J., Greenfield, S., Candy, D., & Geraint, M. (2010). Systematic review: impact of constipation on quality of life in adults and children. *Alimentary Pharmacology and Therapeutics*, Vol. 31, No. 9, pp. 938-949.

Benninga, M., Candy, D.C., Catto-Smith, A.G., Clayden, G., Loening-Baucke, V., Di Lorenzo, C., Nurko, S., & Staiano, A. (2005). The Paris Consensus on Childhood Constipation Terminology (PACCT) Group. *Journal of Pediatric Gastroenterology and Nutrition*, Vol. 40, pp. 273-275.

Boccia, G., Manguso, F., Coccorullo, P., Masi, P., Pensabene, L. & Staiano, A. (2007). Functional Defecation Disorders in Children: PACCT Criteria Versus Rome II Criteria. *Journal of Pediatrics*, Vol. 151, pp. 394-398.

Caplan, A., Walker, L. & Rasquin, A. (2005). Validation of the Pediatric Rome II Criteria for Functional Gastrointestinal Disorders Using the Questionnaire on Pediatric Gastrointestinal Symptoms. *Journal of Pediatric Gastroenterology and Nutrition*, Vol. 41, pp. 305-316.

Catto-Smith, A. (2005). Constipation and toileting issues in children. *Medical Journal of Australia*, Vol. 182, pp. Med J Aust 2005. 182:242-246.

Clarke, M.C., Chow, C.S., Chase, J.W., Gibb, S., Hutson, J.M., & Southwell, B.R. (2008). Quality of life in children with slow transit constipation. *Journal of Pediatric Surgery*, Vol. 43, No. 2, pp. 320-324.

Ho, T. & Caldwell, P. (2008). Management of childhood faecal incontinence. *Medicine Today*, Vol. 9, No. 10, pp. 50-56.

Hyams, J., Colletti, R., Faure, C., Gabriel-Martinez, E., Maffei, H.V., Morais, M.B., Hock, Q.S., & Vandenplas, Y. (2002). Functional gastrointestinal disorders: Working Group Report of the First World Congress of Pediatric Gastroenterology, Hepatology and Nutrition. *Journal of Pediatric Gastroenterology and Nutrition*, Vol. 35, Supp. 2, pp. S110-117.

Hyman, P., Milla, P., Benninga, M., Davidson, G., Fleisher, D. & Taminiau, J. (2006). Childhood Functional Gastrointestinal Disorders: Neonate / Toddler. *Gastroenterology*, Vol. 130, pp. 1519-1526.

Joinson, C., Heron, J., Butler, U., & von Gontard, A. (2006). Psychological differences between children with and without soiling problems (ALSPAC study). *Pediatrics*, Vol. 117, No. 5, pp. 1575–1584.

Levine, M.D. (1975). Children with encopresis: a descriptive analysis. *Pediatrics*, Vol. 56, pp. 412-416.

Lewis, S.J. & Heaton, K.W. (1997). Stool Form Scale as a Useful Guide to Intestinal Transit Time. *Scandinavian Journal of Gastroenterology*, Vol. 32, No. 9, pp. 920-924.

Loening- Baucke, V. (1990). Modulation of abnormal defaecation dynamics by biofeedback treatment in chronically constipated children with encopresis. *Journal of Pediatrics*, Vol. 116, pp. 214-222.

Loening-Baucke, V. (1993). Constipation in early childhood: patient characteristics, treatment, and long-term follow-up. *Gut*, Vol. 34, pp. 1400-1404.

Loening-Baucke, V. (1997). Urinary incontinence and urinary tract infection and their resolution with treatment of chronic constipation of childhood. *Pediatrics*, Vol. 100, No. 2, pp. 228-232.

Loening-Baucke, V. (2004). Functional faecal retention with encopresis in childhood. *Journal of Pediatric Gastroenterology and Nutrition*, Vol. 38, pp. 79-84.

Loening-Baucke, V. & Swidsinski, A. (2007). Constipation as a cause of Acute Abdominal Pain in Children. *Journal of Pediatrics,* Vol. 151, pp. 666-669.

McGrath, K.H., Caldwell, P.H.Y., & Jones, M.P. (2008). The frequency of constipation in children with nocturnal enuresis: a comparison with parental reporting. *Journal of Paediatrics and Child Health,* Vol. 44, pp. 19-27.

Miele, E., Simeone, D., Marino, A., Greco, L., Auricchio, R., Novek, S.J., & Staiano, A. (2004). Functional gastrointestinal disorders in children: an Italian prospective survey. *Pediatrics,* Vol. 114, pp. 73-78.

O'Regan, S., & Yazbeck, S. (1985). Constipation: a cause of enuresis, urinary tract infection and vesico-ureteric reflux in children. *Medical Hypotheses,* Vol. 17, pp. 409-413.

O'Regan, S., Yazbeck, S., Hamberger, B., & Schick, E. (1986). Constipation: a commonly unrecognised cause of enuresis. *American Journal of Diseases in Children,* Vol. 140, pp. 260-261.

Rajindrajith, S., Devanarayana, N., Mettananda, S., Perera, P., Jasmin, S., Karunarathna, U., Adhihetty, D., & Goonewardena, R. (2009). Constipation and functional faecal retention in a group of school children in a district in Sri Lanka. *Sri Lanka Journal of Child Health,* Vol. 38, pp. 60-64.

Rasquin, A., Di Lorenzo, C., Forbes, D., Guiraldes, E., Hyams, J., Staiano, A., & Walker, L. (2006). Childhood Functional Gastrointestinal Disorders: Child / Adolescent. *Gastroenterology,* Vol. 130, pp. 1527-1537.

Rasquin-Weber, A., Hyman, P., Cucchiara, S., Fleisher, D., Hyams, J., Milla, P., Staiano, A. (1999). Childhood functional gastrointestinal disorders. *Gut,* Vol. 45, Supp. 2, pp. 1160-1168.

Saps, M., & Di Lorenzo, C. (2004). Inter-rater reliability of the Rome criteria in children. *Journal of Pediatric Gastroenterology and Nutrition,* Vol. 39, Supp. 1, p S36.

Schurman, J.V., Friesen, C.A., Danda, C.E., Andre, L., Welchert, E., Lavenbarg, T., Cockin, J.T. & Hyman, P.E. (2005). Diagnosing Functional Abdominal Pain with the Rome II Criteria: Parent, Child and Clinician Agreement. *Journal of Pediatric Gastroenterology and Nutrition,* Vol. 41, pp. 291-295.

Taitz, L.S., Water, J.K.H., Urwin, O.M., & Molner, D. (1986). Factors associated with outcome in management of defecation disorders. *Archives of Disease in Childhood,* Vol. 61, pp. 472-477.

van den Berg, M.M., Benninga, M.A., & Di Lorenzo, C. (2006). Epidemiology of childhood constipation: a systematic review. *American Journal of Gastroenterology,* Vol. 101, pp. 2401-2409.

Van Ginkel, R., Reitsma, J.B., Buller, H.A., van Wijk, M.P., Taminiau, J.A., & Benninga, M.A. (2003). Childhood constipation: longitudinal follow-up beyond puberty. *Gastroenterology,* Vol. 125, pp. 357-363.

Weaver, A. & Dobson, P. (2007). An overview of faecal incontinence in children. *Nursing Times,* Vol. 103, No. 47, pp. 40-42.

Whitlock-Morales, A., McKeand, C., DiFilippo, M. & Elitsur, Y. (2007). Diagnosis and treatment of constipation in children: a survey of primary care physicians in West Virginia. *West Virginia Medical Journal,* Vol. 103, No. 4, pp. 14-16.

Youssef, N.N., Langseder, A.L., Verga, B.J., Mones, R.L., & Rosh, J.R. (2005). Chronic childhood constipation is associated with impaired quality of life: a case controlled study. *Journal of Pediatric Gastroenterology and Nutrition,* Vol. 41, No. 1, pp. 56-60.

2

The Role of Diagnostic Tests in Constipation in Children

Anthony G. Catto-Smith and Kathleen H. McGrath
The Royal Children's Hospital, Melbourne
Australia

1. Introduction

The diagnosis of constipation is usually suspected based on the presence of certain symptoms. These may include infrequent passage of stool, stools that are hard or difficult to pass or the presence of faecal incontinence. A careful clinical history and focussed physical examination are often all that is needed to confirm the diagnosis. There are a number of symptom-based classification tools that have been designed for diagnostic use in clinical practice. These classifications have evolved over time but there remains no universally accepted gold standard. The most recently published classification tool is the Rome III classification system.

In certain situations, further diagnostic investigations may be required to confirm the diagnosis or elicit further details to assist in optimal management of the patient. These investigations may range from simple blood tests or abdominal radiography to more complex measures of colonic transit and function that are only available in specialised centres.

This chapter will examine, evaluate and define the role of each of these tests using an evidence based approach. It will determine when it is appropriate to do physiological or other testing in constipated children and assist clinicians in selecting the most appropriate modality of investigation for their patients.

2. Physiology of defaecation

The process of defaecation relies upon a complex interplay between pelvic muscles, muscles of the internal and external anal sphincters and the autonomic and somatic nervous systems.

Faecal matter is moved from the colon into the rectum by peristaltic propagation. The presence of faecal matter in the rectum stretches the rectal wall and the puborectalis and levator ani muscles relax. Distension of the rectum induces a parasympathetic response involving contraction of the rectal walls and relaxation of the internal anal sphincter (recto-anal inhibitory reflex).

When faeces enter the anal canal, anal receptors are activated and the voluntary component of the process is initiated. In an appropriate environment and social situation, the external anal sphincter and puborectalis muscle relax and there is simultaneous contraction of the levator ani, abdominal and diaphragm muscles. At this time, defaecation occurs and faecal matter is evacuated from the body.

In instances where the environment or social situation is unsuitable for defaecation to occur, the external anal sphincter voluntarily remains contracted with the help of the pelvic floor muscles. This occurs for a few seconds until the rectal wall is able to adapt and distend to allow for storage of the additional rectal volume.

Some children may achieve voluntary bowel control around the age of 18 months but there is variability in the age of attainment of complete bowel control. Most children will achieve bladder and bowel control and be toilet trained by the age of 3 years.

3. Physiology of constipation

Some children will have an underlying organic cause for their constipation. These children may be identified by the presence of 'red flag' signs on history taking and examination or characteristic findings on diagnostic investigations. The underlying physiological process will differ based on the individual aetiology e.g. Hirschprung disease is caused by absence of enteric nerves and functional obstruction compared with mechanical obstruction in cases of anal stenosis or atresia.

However, in at least 90% of children, there is no underlying organic cause found for constipation and it is termed 'functional constipation'. Withholding behaviour plays an important role in the development of functional constipation in infants, toddlers and young children. These behaviours can originate from an experience of painful defaecation (e.g. related to passage of hard stools or anal fissures), a lack of regular routine with toileting or environmental factors including unfamiliar bathroom environment associated with time of commencement of school.

Withholding behaviours may manifest as grunting or back arching in infants or clenching of the buttocks and repetitive rocking / fidgeting actions in older children. When stool is withheld, the rectal wall adapts and distends to allow for the storage of faecal material. Over time, stool accumulates in the rectum and larger, harder faecal matter is formed, which is then associated with further pain on attempted defaecation. This cycle of persistent painful defaecation can lead to further retentive posturing and toilet avoidance. With time, increasing rectal distension can result in rectal insensitivity and faecal incontinence with a significant impact on the child's quality of life.

4. The use of diagnostic tests in constipation in adults

A recent review summarised the different diagnostic tests available for use in adult constipation (Rao & Meduri, 2011). Using the available evidence, graded recommendations were given for each diagnostic test. These recommendations were based on the presence and quality of evidence in favour of the test in addition to information on specificity, sensitivity, accuracy and predictive values.

Table 1 summarises these findings.

Key:
Grade A1: Excellent evidence in favour of the test based on high specificity, sensitivity, accuracy and positive predictive values.
Grade B2: Good evidence in favour of the test with some evidence on specificity, sensitivity, accuracy and predictive values.

Grade B3: Fair evidence in favour of the test with some evidence on specificity, sensitivity, accuracy and predictive values.
Grade C: Poor evidence in favour of the test with some evidence on specificity, sensitivity, accuracy and predictive values.

<table>
<tr><th colspan="2">Test</th><th>Evidence</th><th>Recommended Grade</th></tr>
<tr><td colspan="2">Blood tests</td><td>No evidence</td><td>C</td></tr>
<tr><td rowspan="3">Imaging</td><td>Abdominal Xray</td><td>Poor</td><td>C</td></tr>
<tr><td>Barium enema</td><td>Poor</td><td>C</td></tr>
<tr><td>Defecography</td><td>Fair</td><td>B3</td></tr>
<tr><td colspan="2">Anorectal Ultrasound</td><td>Poor</td><td>C</td></tr>
<tr><td colspan="2">Magnetic Resonance Imaging</td><td>Fair</td><td>B3</td></tr>
<tr><td colspan="2">Flexible sigmoidoscopy and colonoscopy</td><td>Poor</td><td>C</td></tr>
<tr><td rowspan="3">Gastrointestinal transit studies</td><td>Colonic transit with radiopaque markers</td><td>Good</td><td>B2</td></tr>
<tr><td>Colonic transit with scintigraphy</td><td>Good</td><td>B2</td></tr>
<tr><td>Wireless motility capsule</td><td>Excellent</td><td>A1</td></tr>
<tr><td rowspan="2">Manometric studies</td><td>Anorectal manometry</td><td>Good</td><td>B2</td></tr>
<tr><td>Colonic manometry</td><td>Good</td><td>B2</td></tr>
</table>

Table 1. Summary of diagnostic tests and their recommended grade in adults (modified from Rao & Meduri, 2011).

Table 1 illustrates the variability in the quality of evidence supporting the use of investigations in the diagnosis of adult constipation. In practice, the diagnosis of constipation still relies heavily on careful history-taking and detailed clinical examination technique.

To date, there are limited studies assessing the role of diagnostic tests in constipation in children. A review by Baker and colleagues in 1999graded the quality of evidence for limited investigations in children using methods of the Canadian Preventive Services Task Force. They found that the evidence for abdominal radiography, when interpreted carefully was II-2 (*evidence obtained from well-designed cohort or case-control analytic studies, preferably more than one centre or research group). The evidence for rectal biopsy and rectal manometry in reliable exclusion of Hirschprung disease was II-1 (evidence obtained from well-designed cohort or case-control trials without randomisation). Measurement of transit time using radiopaque markers was graded as II-2* (Baker et al., 1999).

There is limited availability of a supportive consensus guideline for choice of diagnostic tests in children with constipation. This makes the selection of investigations and their interpretation a challenge for many clinicians. This chapter aims to assess the data available with particular focus on the paediatric population group. It outlines both the benefits and limitations of each individual technique to allow clinicians to make an informed decision about when to employ their use.

5. The role of radiography

5.1 Abdominal radiography

The diagnosis of constipation is usually a clinical decision based on good history-taking and physical examination of the child. In clinical practice, abdominal radiography is still performed by some clinicians as part of their initial diagnostic assessment or as a tool to assess and monitor treatment response. There may be a role for abdominal radiography in certain circumstances and these will be discussed below.

Abdominal radiography may be indicated when the diagnosis of chronic constipation is strongly suspected but in doubt because of a lack of supportive evidence on history or examination. In particular, supportive physical signs (in the form of palpable abdominal faecal masses) may be difficult to elicit in obese children or children who have been frequently using stool softeners. Faecal impaction can be suspected clinically and is usually able to be confirmed by rectal examination. However, there may be exceptions where despite a strong suspicion of chronic constipation, there is no palpable faecal retention on rectal examination. The clinical practice guideline of the North American Society for Pediatric Gastroenterology and Nutrition recommends the use of a plain abdominal radiograph for diagnosing constipation in cases where there is uncertainty about the presence of constipation.

Rectal examination is an invasive procedure. Consequently, in some children it may be contraindicated (e.g. in the presence of a history of previous sexual abuse or by the degree of associated psychological distress and angst it causes the child). In these children there may be a role for abdominal radiography in place of a rectal examination to confirm faecal impaction and exclude bowel obstruction prior to the commencement of bowel washout.

Abdominal radiography can be employed in the different circumstances described above. It may also be useful to give a measure of megarectum. The benefits of abdominal radiography include that it is an easily accessible, non-invasive and relatively inexpensive investigation. However, this modality does have some limitations that need to be factored in when it is being considered. Every radiograph performed provides the child with a small dose of ionizing radiation. In isolation, this is unlikely to have direct impact on their wellbeing, but cumulative doses of radiation may be potentially harmful for an individual's health.

The interpretation of abdominal radiography is variable. It has traditionally been largely subjective and open to individual interpretation. In an attempt to objectify the classification of this tool, a number of different scoring systems have been created including the Leech and Barr scoring systems. The Leech score assesses the large intestine in 3 segments: right colon, left colon and rectosigmoid colon and provides a score from 0 to 5 for each segment based on the amount of faeces present (0= no faeces visible to 5= severe faecal loading with bowel dilatation). An overall score out of 15 is obtained, with a score of 9 or greater being positive for constipation. The Barr score divides the large intestine into 4 segments: ascending colon, transverse colon, descending colon and rectum. It quantifies both the amount and consistency of the faeces (e.g. granular, rock-like) and gives a score out of 22 with a score of 10 or greater being positive for constipation (Pensabene et al., 2010).

Despite these formalised classification systems, studies comparing different scoring methods show that there is still a degree of inter-observer variability. This applies to interpretation by both paediatric clinicians and radiologists. Overall, individual scoring systems used for interpretation of faecal loading on abdominal radiograph have a low sensitivity (Pensabene et al., 2010).

A recent systematic review assessed the relationship between clinical symptoms and signs of constipation and the presence of faecal loading on abdominal radiography. The availability of good quality literature was limited, however the study concluded that conflicting evidence exists for an association between the clinical and radiographic diagnosis of constipation. The high quality studies that were assessed in the review found that a radiographic diagnosis of constipation occurs almost as often in clinically constipated children as in clinically non-constipated children. Furthermore, they found that the results of rectal examination were not consistently associated with the presence of fecal retention on abdominal radiography. The review concluded that there is inadequate evidence to support the North American Society for Pediatric Gastroenterology and Nutrition clinical practice guideline and those clinicians who recommend a plain abdominal radiograph in cases of uncertainty of the presence of constipation in a child (Reuchlin-Vroklage LM et al., 2005).

There is a clear need for further clinical research to assess the precise role of abdominal radiography in the diagnosis of constipation in children. Current data provides conflicting opinion and challenging interpretation for clinicians. A better availability of future quality literature shall help to determine the indications for this investigation and validate its use in clinical practice.

5.2 Contrast radiography

5.2.1 Barium enema

A barium enema (lower gastrointestinal series) is a diagnostic procedure where opaque contrast medium (barium sulfate) is infused into the colon via a rectal enema tube. The flow of barium sulfate is captured by using fluoroscope xray pictures. The patient may be asked to move into different positions to obtain optimal detailed anatomical images of the gastrointestinal tract.

Barium enema can be useful in some instances for the identification of anatomical abnormalities including megacolon, megarectum or rectal masses. It may also be used as an initial screening for Hirschsprung's Disease (a condition characterised by the absence of ganglion cells in the myenteric plexus of the distal colon). The visualisation of a transition radiographic zone and delayed barium emptying is suggestive of Hirschsprung's Disease however not diagnostic. A rectal biopsy is still required to confirm this diagnosis. In neonates, the absence of a transition zone may be a normal variant making this test less useful in this particular age group.

Limitations associated with this modality include associated radiation exposure and the invasive nature of the procedure (requiring placement of an enema tube into the rectum).

Barium enema has little or no role as a routine investigation in the workup of children with chronic constipation but may be used to assess gastrointestinal anatomy in some patients.

5.2.2 Defaecating proctography

Defaecating proctography assesses the mechanics of defaecation in real time using fluoroscopy. A barium paste is manually infused into the rectum using specialised equipment until there is adequate distension. The patient then moves to a portable plastic commode and their process of defaecation is recorded by an x-ray camera.

Defaecating proctography is not commonly performed in current practice. It may have a limited role in assessment of pelvic floor dysfunction (including anismus) in obstructed defaecation. Its main limitations include associated radiation exposure and invasive nature of the procedure.

6. The role of blood tests

Any child undergoing assessment for chronic functional or intractable constipation should have certain blood tests done to exclude an underlying organic cause. This is particularly the case where there are clinical signs or symptoms present that are suggestive of an underlying metabolic or pathological process.

Patients should undergo a complete blood count and biochemical profile, in particular looking at serum calcium levels to exclude hypercalcemia and blood glucose levels to look for evidence of diabetes. Thyroid function tests should be done to exclude hypothyroidism and a coeliac screen and total IgA to assess for evidence of coeliac disease. A diagnosis of coeliac disease can only be confirmed by endoscopy and small intestinal biopsy.

Less commonly, measurement of blood lead levels may be indicated to exclude lead toxicity as an aetiological factor.

7. The role of ultrasound

Ultrasound scan is a safe, non invasive and easily accessible mode of imaging. It is not currently widely utilised in children with constipation, but has a potential role in quantifying the degree of faecal loading / megarectum and monitoring of treatment response.

7.1 Pelvic ultrasound

Pelvic ultrasound scan can be used to visualise faeces of both hard and soft consistency. One group in the United Kingdom have successfully used pelvic ultrasound together with a scoring system in their outpatient management of constipated children since 2007 (Lakshminarayanan B et al., 2008). Their findings showed that the presence of faecal loading on ultrasound correlated highly with clinical symptoms of constipation on history taking. In addition, of the 269 patients (54%) with no palpable faeces on clinical abdominal examination, 31% of them showed significant faecal loading on ultrasound. This finding supports the notion that despite a thorough history and physical examination, some patients with constipation may still be missed. In patients in whom there remains an ongoing clinical suspicion of constipation, there may be a role for investigations such as ultrasound scan. Lakshminarayanan and colleagues successfully illustrated the use of this modality to diagnose and monitor treatment response of their patients in outpatient clinical practice.

Other studies have attempted to quantify the degree of constipation by using rectal diameter and other measurements on ultrasound scan (Karaman et al., 2010; Joensson et al., 2008). These groups found that a thicker mean rectal diameter correlated with a clinical diagnosis of constipation by Rome III criteria. Furthermore, they found that the amount of faecal loading on ultrasound decreased by a significant amount after one month of treatment supporting a role for this modality in monitoring of treatment response.

Karaman and colleagues could identify no inter-observer difference between 2 different radiologists performing the ultrasound scans. This supports a degree of reliability between different users of ultrasound scan as an imaging modality. Further detailed studies to assess for inter-observer differences between paediatric clinicians and radiologists interpreting ultrasound in this context would be useful.

Pelvic ultrasound is appropriate for use in the outpatient setting. It has no associated radiation dose. It is a non-invasive procedure and in the hands of experienced staff, tends to be well tolerated by children. There are only limited studies available on the use of pelvic ultrasound in constipated children and further research would be beneficial to help ascertain the precise role for this modality in the assessment and long term monitoring of this patient group.

7.2 Endoanal ultrasound

Endoanal ultrasound involves insertion of an ultrasound probe into the anus allowing visualisation of the internal sphincter, external sphincter and puborectalis muscles. It can be used to provide information about the anatomical course of anal fistulae and some anal abscesses.

Endoanal ultrasound is relatively quick and simple to perform. There is no associated radiation dose. In some children it may not be well tolerated due to its invasive nature and may require the use of sedation or general anaesthetic in order to perform effectively. In addition, patients must undergo an enema a few hours beforehand to ensure adequate clearance of the rectal area prior to scanning.

8. The role of gastrointestinal transit studies

Colonic transit studies have traditionally provided information about total and segmental colonic transit time and overall colorectal motor function. There are 2 standard techniques performed: radio-opaque marker studies and radio-nuclide scintigraphy. Both techniques give similar information for ascending and transverse colon motility but radio-opaque marker studies generally produce faster total transit time (Southwell et al., 2009).

Colonic transit studies classify children with constipation into 3 subgroups:

1. Children with normal colonic transit time
2. Children with outlet obstruction
3. Children with slow transit constipation.

Colonic transit studies can be used to differentiate slow-transit constipation from pelvic dyssynergia. In clinical practice, this information can be useful to identify patients with motility disorders including Hirschsprung's disease and chronic intestinal pseudo-obstruction. It can also be used to help differentiate children with functional constipation and overflow incontinence from those with nonretentive faecal incontinence (Benninga et al. 1994). This is important as management differs between the two conditions.

Colonic transit studies may also have a role in predicting patient prognosis. One study showed a colon transit time of > 100 hours was associated with a poor treatment outcome at one year (de Lorijn et al., 2004). The range of normal colonic transit is 20-56 hours and there is little variation between children and adults (Southwell et al., 2009).

A more recent innovation is the use of wireless capsule technology. The additional benefits of radio-nuclide scintigraphy and wireless capsule monitoring are their capacity to give information about gastrointestinal transit in the stomach and small intestine as well as the colon. In cases of severe refractory constipation, this data may be useful in pre-operative assessment to aid decision-making about the portion of bowel for resection and the best position(s) for stoma creation. Information on gastric and small intestinal motility may also be useful in children with abnormal gastric emptying to help decide on appropriate methods of feeding (e.g. gastrostomy versus jejunostomy feeds).

8.1 Radio-opaque marker studies

This technique was first pioneered in adults in the late 1960s. There are a number of variations in its application including a few more commonly used methods. Firstly, there is the 'simple' radio-opaque marker test where a single capsule is swallowed (containing 20-50 markers) and a single abdominal radiograph is taken 4-5 days later showing the location of the markers. Alternatively, a single capsule (containing multiple markers) is ingested and radiographs are performed every 24 hours until the markers are no longer visible. A third technique is the 'multiple markers' test where a single capsule is ingested daily for 3 days (each containing a different shaped marker) and abdominal radiographs are taken at days 4 and 7 after ingestion. The different marker shapes help to identify their individual locations.

Delayed transit is defined as retention of more than 20% of markers at the time of abdominal radiograph (96 hours for the 'simple' test and 120 hours for the 'multiple markers' test) (Dinning and Di Lorenzo, 2011). Children should refrain from taking laxatives in the weeks before the study as these may affect bowel function and subsequent results.

Radio-opaque marker studies are inexpensive, relatively widely available and are useful in the identification of slow transit constipation. Their downside is the associated variability with the use of different methodologies and the lack of information gained regarding transit in the rest of the gastrointestinal tract.

8.2 Radio-nuclide scintigraphy

Radio-nuclide scintigraphy has been utilised since the mid 1980s. It involves oral ingestion of a labelled isotope followed by gamma camera scans at various intervals up to 5 days (depending on the specific method used). The progression of the isotope throughout colonic regions is plotted using graphs. It is possible to calculate the amount of isotope residue at each region for each time interval. Various measures of isotope retention can be used to diagnose and quantify delayed colonic transit. There include transit time in hours, % radioactivity retained, proximal colonic emptying and centre of mass.

Radio-nuclide scintigraphy is expensive and requires an appropriately equipped and trained specialist centre which may not be readily accessible to all clinicians. In addition, results of different studies may not be directly comparable due to differences in the method of isotope administration (e.g. liquid verus solid markers) and varying measurements of interpretation used. However, radio-nuclide scintigraphy can be useful for classification of pathophysiological subtypes of constipation as outlined in the introduction to section 6.

8.3 Wireless capsule technology

This is a relatively recent innovation. It involves an ingestible gastrointestinal capsule, a receiver worn by the patient during the study period, a receiver docking station and display software. The capsule is able to identify and transmit information about intraluminal pH, pressure and temperature and has a battery life of 5 days.

To date, there are no large studies looking at the use of wireless capsule technology in children and little clinical experience from clinical application in this population group. Limited research available in adult patients has compared wireless capsule assessment of gastrointestinal motility with radio-nuclide scintigraphy. A recent study performed simultaneous whole gut scintigraphy and wireless capsule monitoring of whole gut transit in 10 adults. They found a very strong correlation between measurements of gastric emptying by the two different methods (Maqbool et al, 2009).

Potential benefits of this technique include no associated radiation exposure and its capacity to provide information about stomach and small intestine transit as well as colonic transit (by its ability to monitor pH and thus detect progression from the stomach into the small intestine).

In children, this technique may have some limitations. It relies upon the ingestion of a wireless capsule which some younger children may find difficult or unappealing. An alternative option is placement of the capsule into the stomach at the time of an endoscope.

This technique is relatively new to clinical practice and further studies are needed to elucidate its precise role in the investigation of children with constipation.

9. Manometric studies

Manometry involves the measurement of pressures in various segments of the gastrointestinal tract to provide information on gastrointestinal function and motility. Both water perfused and solid state catheters have been used.

9.1 Anorectal manometry

Anorectal manometry assesses the motor function of the anal sphincters, sensory thresholds to rectal distension, recto-anal inhibitory reflexes and coordination of evacuation. Some degree of bowel preparation is required beforehand. A transducer is inserted through the anus with the child in the left lateral position and a sphincter pressure profile measured. Transient inflation of a balloon at the tip of the catheter assembly allows measurement of sensory thresholds, and also confirms normal reflex relaxation of the internal anal sphincter (rectoanal inhibitory reflex). Attempted evacuation of the rectal balloon allows examination of the normal coordination of evacuation as well as the response to withholding (squeezing).

Anorectal manometry is useful to exclude sphincteric damage, and rule out Hirschsprung disease. Blunted sensation to rectal distension and megarectum can also be defined.

Anorectal manometry also has a role in the identification of dyssynergic defaecation and altered rectal sensation in children with constipation (Rao et al., 2011). The normal process of defaecation involves relaxation of the puborectalis muscle and external anal sphincter combined with an adequate propulsive force. Pelvic floor dyssynergia occurs when there is abnormal pelvic floor muscle relaxation or even paradoxical contraction during the process of attempted defaecation. These children are unable to produce the coordination required for normal defaecation and frequently become constipated.

Identification of dyssynergic defaecation is important as it changes management intervention. These children do not require laxative management but will benefit from behavioural interventions and possibly from the use of biofeedback therapy (Chiarioni et al., 2006). Biofeedback therapy is a method of neuromuscular re-education. A computer and video monitor are used to display bodily processes to a patient that they are normally unaware of. Increased awareness of these behaviours provides an opportunity to consciously modify one's responses to a more acceptable pattern.

The most common problem associated with the use of anorectal manometry is that it is limited to certain specialised centres. Other complications may include a lack of standardisation in technique between different transducers and technical errors related to inadequate balloon sufflation or positioning (Benninga et al., 2004).

Anorectal manometry provides information on pathophysiological abnormalities underlying childhood constipation.

9.1.1 Rectal barostat test

The rectal barostat test consists of a highly compliant balloon placed in the rectum and connected to a barostat (computerised pressure-distending device). This device is able to record detailed information on tone, compliance and assess rectal sensation.

The information obtained by this technique can be useful in identification of megarectum, hyper- or hypo- compliant rectum. Rectal compliance, sensation and function are all closely inter-related.

9.2 Colonic manometry

Colonic manometry provides a detailed picture of overall motor activity of the colon. The American Neurogastroenterology and Motility Society recently recommended its use in assessment of severely constipated children unresponsive to medical therapy, with evidence of slow colonic transit and the absence of an evacuatory disorder (Camilleri et al., 2008). It can be also be used to differentiate functional constipation from constipation secondary to an underlying neuromuscular cause.

On study looked at the indications for colonic manometry in a group of 146 children referred to a tertiary centre in the USA (Pensabene et al., 2003). The 4 main indications identified for use of colonic manometry were:

1. Clarification of pathophysiology of lower gastrointestinal symptoms (68%)
2. Clarification of pathophysiology of persisting lower gastrointestinal symptoms after surgery for Hirschsprung's Disease (14%)

3. Confirmation of diagnosis of intestinal pseudo-obstruction (11%)
4. Assistance with decision about re-anastomosis of a diverted colon (7%).

Colonic manometry is performed by using colonic catheters that incorporate multiple recording ports or sensors. These provide a feedback of information on intraluminal pressures to a recording system. The catheters can be water-perfused or solid state, with most paediatric centres favouring the former (Dinning PG & Di Lorenzo C, 2011). Catheters are usually placed by colonoscope or via radiological guidance such as fluoroscopy after adequate colonic clearance using bowel preparation. They can be placed into the mouth, nose, anus (most common) or through an existing stoma. The study period generally lasts around 5 hours but may be up to 24 hours in duration.

Water-perfused catheters consist of flexible tubing with multiple recording ports connected to a pneumohydraulic infusion pump that provides a constant flow of water. Colonic wall contractions occlude the ports and impede water flow and this resistance to flow is transmitted as pressure change to external transducers. These catheters are relatively cost effective and some are autoclaveable and re-usable. On the downside, patients are confined to bed for the duration of the study and uncertainty exists regarding whether large amounts of infused water may have deleterious effects in young children (Dinning et al., 2010).

Solid-state catheters comprise strain gauges embedded into a flexible tube. Each gauge connects to a recording system by fine wiring. Used with portable recorders, these catheters allow the patient to be ambulant because they don't rely on constant water flow. However they do tend to be more expensive than water-perfused catheters (Dinning et al., 2010).

There are 2 types of normal colonic motor activity:
1. Low- amplitude tonic and phasic contractions (mixing of luminal contents)
2. High-amplitude propagated contractions (propulsion of stool from colon to rectum).

In addition, colonic motility should increase after a meal (gastro-colonic response) and respond to other physiological stimuli such as morning waking and exercise (Hussain SZ & Di Lorenzo C, 2002). The presence of these features of normal colonic motility in the context of constipation suggests a behavioural cause or functional constipation.

In the case of abnormalities, colonic manometry can distinguish between an underlying neuropathy and myopathy. Weak or absent colonic contractions in the absence of generalised colonic dilatation suggests a colonic myopathy. Absent, disordered or abnormal colonic contractions combined with an absent gastro-colonic meal response suggests the presence of an underlying neuropathy.

Colonic manometry may also have a role in monitoring of treatment response in constipation management. A study by Pensabene et al in 2003 showed that the results of colonic manometry resulted in recommendations to adjust management plans (mostly surgical intervention) in 93% of 146 children. Of the 98 patients that were able to be contacted for follow up data, 88% had parents who believed that these interventions had been a positive impact on their child's health.

Colonic manometry is a useful diagnostic tool in childhood chronic constipation and a number of international centres are trained in this technique. Compared with adults, there are less underlying systemic diseases or drugs affecting colonic motility in children and the results tend to be easier to interpret in this younger population.

Limitations related to this diagnostic procedure include variation related to use of different catheter types, placement techniques and protocols in different centres. It is also associated with a degree of invasiveness and so may not be tolerated well by some children.

10. Electromyography

Electromyography records the electrical activity of skeletal muscles and can be used to assess for evidence of abnormal skeletal muscle function. Combined with manometry, it can be useful to confirm the presence of paradoxical sphincteric contraction during attempted defaecation.

11. The role of biopsy

The most common biopsy performed in relation to childhood constipation is a rectal biopsy. This is done in cases of suspected Hirschsprung's disease to confirm a diagnosis. The child may or may not have had other previous investigations including barium enema or anal manometry.

Usually a suction-method biopsy is performed. This is a simple and quick procedure, though does carry a risk for haemorrhage. In neonates, it can be performed at the bedside without the need for a general anaesthetic. Occasionally there may be difficulty obtaining an adequate tissue specimen by this technique (as it is a blind procedure). In these circumstances, a full thickness surgical biopsy may need to be performed.

There may be a role for other gastrointestinal tract biopsies to demonstrate abnormal histology in the presence of chronic constipation (e.g. neuronal intestinal dysplasia: qualitative and quantitative abnormalities of the myenteric plexus).

12. Magnetic Resonance Imaging

Magnetic resonance imaging (MRI) of the spine may be performed in children with constipation if the patient history or physical examination is suggestive of spinal pathology. A recent study looked at the result of MRI-spine scans performed on 88 children with intractable constipation. They found that 9% (8 children) had spinal abnormalities on MRI that required surgery (75% of these were a tethered cord). Of these 8 children, 5 had no abnormal signs on physical examination. (Rosen et al., 2004). This study highlights the importance of a thorough history and physical examination in any child presenting with chronic constipation. In particular, one should assess the lower limb neurological status and sacral area for any abnormalities (skin discolouration, naevi, sinuses, hairy patch, central pit or bony abnormalities).

MRI and MR defecography (dynamic pelvic MRI) have also been used in the assessment of anorectal disorders. They have the advantage of being able to simultaneously image anatomy and motility function and a low dosage of radiation exposure. However, there is a high associated cost and very limited data exists on the role of this investigation in children.

13. Miscellaneous Investigations

There are some other investigations that may be indicated in assessment for underlying causes in chronic constipation. These include the following:

1. Sweat test to exclude cystic fibrosis. In particular, this condition may be suspected in cases of constipation associated with failure to thrive, recurrent chest infections or a history of delayed passage of meconium or meconium plug.
2. Allergy testing (IgE antibodies to cow's milk protein antigens) for cow's milk protein allergy. This may be suspected in the context of constipation if the patient has a strong history of allergies, anal fissures / excoriation or abdominal discomfort.

14. Conclusion

Most children with chronic constipation do not require any investigations other than a thorough history and physical examination. In patients with intractable constipation or red flags suggestive of an underlying organic aetiology, specialised testing may be indicated and of use. The choice of investigations should be made with specific consideration to the diagnosis being considered.

15. References

Baker, S.S., Liptak, G.S., Colletti, R.B., Croffie, J.M., Di Lorenzo, C., Ector, W. & Nurko, S. (1999). Constipation in infants and children: evaluation and treatment: a medical position statement of the North American Society for Pediatric Gastroenterology and Nutrition. *Journal of Pediatric Gastroenterlogy and Nutrition,* Vol. 29, No. 5, pp. 612-626.

Benninga, M.A., Buller, H.A., Heymans, H.A.S., Tytgat, G.N.J. & Taminiau, J.A.J.M. (1994). Is encopresis always the result of constipation? *Archives of Diseases in Childhood,* Vol. 71, pp. 186-193.

Benninga, M.A., Büller, H.A., Staalman, C.R., Gubler, F.M., Bossuyt, P.M., van der Plas, R.N., & Taminiau, J.A.J.M. (1995). Defaecation disorders in children, colonic transit time versus the Barr-score. *European Journal of Pediatrics,* Vol.154, No. 4, pp. 277-284.

Benninga, M., Voskuijl, W. & Taminau, J. (2004). Childhood Constipation: Is there new light in the tunnel? *Journal of Paediatric Gastroenterology and Nutrition,* Vol.39, pp. 448-464.

Bewley, A., Clancy, M.J., & Hall, J.R. (1989). The erroneous use by an accident and emergency department of plain abdominal radiographs in the diagnosis of constipation. *Archives of Emergency Medicine,* Vol. 6, pp. 257-258.

Blethyn, A.J., Verrier Jones, K., Newcombe, R., Roberts, G.M., & Jenkins, H.R. (1995). Radiological assessment of constipation. *Archives of Diseases in Childhood,* Vol. 73, pp. 532-533.

Camilleri, M., Bharucha, A.E., Di Lorenzo, C., Hasler, W.L., Prather, C.M., Rao, S.S., & Wald, A. (2008). American Neurogastroenterology and Motility Society consensus statement on intraluminal measurement of gastrointestinal and colonic motility in clinical practice. *Neurogastroenterology and Motility,* Vol. 29, pp. 1269-1282.

Chiarioni, G., Heymen, S., & Whitehead, W.E. (2006). Biofeedback therapy for dyssynergic defecation. World Journal of Gastroenterology. Vol 12, pp 7069-7074.

de Lorijn, F., van Wijk, M.P., Reitsma, J.B., van Ginkel, R., Taminiau, J.A., & Benninga, M.A. (2004). Prognosis of constipation: clinical factors and colonic transit time. *Archives of Diseases in Childhood,* Vol. 89, pp. 723-727.

Dinning, P.G., Benninga, M.A., Southwell, B.R. & Scott, S.M. (2010). Paediatric and adult colonic manometry: A tool to help unravel the pathophysiology of constipation. *World Journal of Gastroenterology,* Vol. 16, No. 41, pp. 5162-5172.

Dinning, P.G. & Di Lorenzo, C. (2011). Colonic dysmotility in constipation. *Best Practice and Research Clinical Gastroenterology,* Vol. 25, pp. 89-101.

Hussain, S.Z., & Di Lorenzo, C. (2002). Motility disorders, diagnosis and treatment for the paediatric patient. *Pediatric Clinics of North America,* Vol. 49, No.1, pp. 27-51.

Joensson, I.M., Siggaard, C., Rittig, S., Hagstroem, S. & Djurhus, J.C. (2008). Transabdominal ultrasound of rectum as a diagnostic tool in childhood constipation. *Journal of Urology,* Vol. 179, No. 5, pp. 1997-2002.

Karaman, A., Ramadan, S., Karaman, I., Gokharman, D., Erdogan, D., Kacar, M., Cavusoglu, Y., & Kosar, U. (2010). Diagnosis and follow-up in constipated children: should we use ultrasound? *Journal of Pediatric Surgery,* Vol. 45, No. 9, pp. 1849-1855.

Leech, S.C., McHugh, K., & Sullivan, P.B. (1999). Evaluation of a method of assessing faecal loading on plain abdominal radiographs in children. *Pediatric Radiology,* Vol. 29, pp. 255-258.

Maqbool, S., Parkman, H.P. & Friedenberg, F.K. (2009). Wireless capsule motility: Comparison of the Smartpill GI monitoring system with scinitigraphy for measuring whole gut transit. *Digestive Diseases and Sciences,* Vol. 54, pp. 2167-2174.

Meunier, P., Marechal, J.M., & Mollard, P. (1978). Accuracy of the manometric diagnosis of Hirschsprung's disease. *Journal of Pediatric Surgery,* Vol. 13, pp. 411-415.

Nurko, S.S. (2004). Gastrointestinal manometer. Methodology indications. In Walker, W.A. et al., (Eds). (2004). *Paediatric Gastrointestinal Disease,* B.C. Decker Inc.: Philadelphia, pp. 1786-1808.

Nurko, S. (2005). What's the value of diagnostic tools in defecation disorders? *Journal of Pediatric Gastroenterology and Nutrition,* Vol. 41, pp. S53-55.

Papadopoulou, A., Clayden, G.S., & Booth, I.W. (1994). The clinical value of solid marker transit studies in childhood constipation and soiling. *European Journal of Pediatrics,* Vol. 153,pp. 560-564.

Pensabene, L., Buonomo, C., Fishman, L., Chitkara, D. & Nurko, S. (2010). Lack of utility of abdominal x-rays in the evaluation of children with constipation: comparison of different scoring methods. *Journal of Pediatric Gastroenterology and Nutrition,* Vol. 51, No. 2, pp. 155-159.

Pensabene, L., Youssef, N.N., Griffiths, J.M., & Di Lorenzo, C. (2003). Colonic manometry in children with defecatory disorders: role in diagnosis and management. *American Journal of Gastroenterology,* Vol. 98, No.5, pp. 1052-1057.

Rao, S.S.C. and Meduri, K. (2011). What is necessary to diagnose constipation? *Best Practice and Research Clinical Gastroenterology,* Vol. 25, pp. 127-140.

Reuchlin-Vroklage, L.M., Bierma-Zeinstra, S., Benninga, M.A., & Berger, M.Y. (2005). Diagnostic value of abdominal radiography in constipated children: a systematic review. *Archives of Pediatrics and Adolescent Medicine,* Vol. 159, pp. 671-678.

Rosen, R., Buonomo, C., Andrade, R., & Nurko, S. (2004). Incidence of spinal cord lesions in patients with intractable constipation. *Journal of Pediatrics,* Vol. 145, pp. 409-411.

Southwell, B.R., Clarke, M.C.C., Sutcliffe, J. & Hutson, J.M. (2009). Colonic transit studies: normal values for adults and children with comparison of radiological and scintigraphic methods. *Pediatric Surgery International,* Vol. 25, pp. 559-572.

3

The Role of Interstitial Cells of Cajal (ICC) in Gastrointestinal Motility Disorders – What the Gastroenterologist Has to Know

Christian Breuer
Clinic of General Pediatrics,
Department of Pediatric Gastroenterology,
University Children's Hospital Hamburg-Eppendorf,
Germany

1. Introduction

Undisturbed gastrointestinal motility or peristalsis is critical for effective digestion and absorption of our food and its ingredients. Peristaltic waves in the gut are propelled by the circular and longitudinal layers of smooth muscle cells in the different segments of the gastrointestinal tract. The initiation and regulation of peristalsis is a complex process which, secondary to smooth muscle cells and enteric nerves, involves pacemaker cells of mesenchymal origin called interstitial cells of Cajal (ICC).

ICC form a network, which is widely distributed in all layers of the gastrointestinal tract. In recent years, there is growing evidence that ICC serve as electrical pacemakers and generate spontaneous electrical slow waves which constitute the basic electrical rhythm in the gastrointestinal tract. Additionally, they are important for the active propagation of slow waves and mediate neurotransmission between inhibitory and excitatory enteric neurons and smooth muscle cells.

Despite their first description more than 100 years ago, only in recent years their importance for the regulation of smooth muscle activity has been discovered. By now the presence of ICC or ICC-like cells has been demonstrated in most visceral organs which generate spontaneous rhythmic muscle contractions, e.g. the urinary and genital system.

The foremost aim of this chapter will be to inform the reader about the recent insights in the role of ICC for the physiologic course of gastrointestinal motility. A short overview about anatomical morphology, signal transduction, physiology and function will be given.

Until recently only little was known about the relevance of ICC as a pathogenetic factor for specific gastrointestinal motility diseases. By now, loss or dysfunction of ICC networks has been associated with slow transit constipation, idiopathic megacolon, diabetic gastropathy, and other diseases of impaired gastrointestinal motility. This chapter will give a short overview about the recent knowledge and highlight the role of ICC in the pathogenesis of gastrointestinal motility disorders.

2. History and morphology of interstitial cells of Cajal and the ICC network

Long lasting constipation is a common problem for up to 10% of the population in the western world. Especially children and elderly people are affected. The symptom of constipation can be the result of many different anatomical, metabolic or functional disorders. For decades physicians and scientists saw the interaction between the enteric nerve system and the smooth muscle cells of the gut as the central point for regulation of sound peristalsis, facilitating proper segmentation and absorption of food and nutrients. Only during the last two decades it became obvious, that the core unit that controls gastrointestinal motility also includes ICC.

For more than 100 years ICC have been known to the histologists as mesenchymal cells ubiquitously distributed within the tunica muscularis of the bowel. The later Nobel prize laureate Santiago Ramón y Cajal first described the cells that are located *interstitially* between nerve endings and smooth muscle cells (Cajal, 1893). They form a network, which is found in all layers of the gastrointestinal tract. They represent approximately 5% of cells that make up the tunica muscularis and develop independently of neuronal crest-derived enteric neurons or glia from mesenchymal precursor cells. Although we know almost nothing about the metabolism, differentiation, and regeneration of these cells, a dense, comprehensive network of these spindle-shaped cells can be found in the newborn as well as in elderly people.

The distribution of ICC varies between the different layers and different segments of the gastrointestinal tract. Myenteric ICC (ICC-MY) form dense networks and are closely located to the myenteric plexus between the circular and longitudinal layers of the tunica muscularis. More loosely scattered ICC are found in the deep muscular plexus (ICC-DMP) and even in the submucosa of the stomach and colon. Intramuscular ICC within the circular and longitudinal layers of muscle in the gastrointestinal tract (ICC-IM) are closely associated with nerve varicosities throughout the muscularis propria. The tight contact of ICC with nerve cell varicosities and smooth muscle cells prompted theories they might conduct signal transmission between the gastrointestinal nerve system and smooth muscle cells. Already Ramón y Cajal himself suspected their involvement in transduction of nerve impulses after recognizing the close associations between ICC, enteric neurons, and smooth muscle cells. He used methylene blue stains when he characterized the cells at the beginning of the twentieth century so well, that they still bear his name (Cajal, 1911).

Typical ICC are defined through their spindle-shaped, elongated body with several branches and processes. The nucleus is ovoid and a basal lamina and a thick capsula made of collagen may envelope the cells (Faussone-Pellegrini and Thuneberg, 1999). With the support of modern electron microscopy more ultrastructural details of these cells have been defined and they could now be divided into at least three different types by comparing their intracellular characteristics. These include abundant mitochondria, endoplasmatic reticulum and intermediate filaments, whereas contractile proteins are missing. Frequent gap junctions are seen between the ICC to form the network through the bowel wall (Streutker et al., 2007).

In recent years the search for different specific markers for ICC has resulted in a rapidly increasing number of approaches applicable for light and fluorescence microscopy. The new interest in ICC increased rapidly twenty years ago, when Hitomi Maeda established an easy-to-use marker protein for ICC, identifying ICC as Kit-expressing cells using an anti-Kit antibody (Maeda et al., 1992). The protein encoded by *c-kit* is the receptor tyrosin kinase Kit

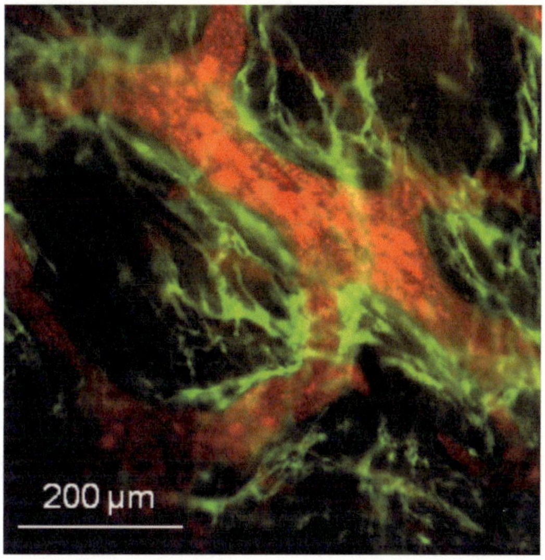

Fig. 1. Normal morphology of c-Kit stained ICC and PGP-positive myenteric neurons in human ileum. Note the dense network of ICC linked by many branches and processes overlying the myenteric ganglion (staining for the neuronal marker PGP 9.5, red; PH164, The Binding Site, Birmingham, UK; staining for c-Kit, green; PC34, Oncogene, Boston, MA, USA).

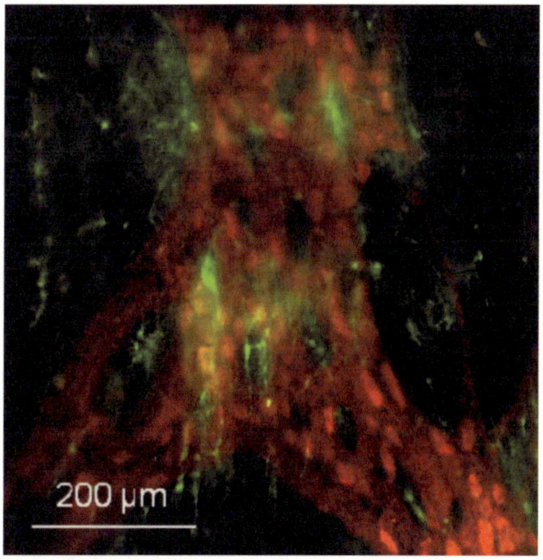

Fig. 2. Abnormal morphology of myenteric ICC and enteric neurons in the colonic biopsy of an adolescent with slow transit constipation. Note the reduced density and ramification of the ICC network. Also remarkable are the gaps in the ganglion structure, which are highly uncommon in young patients.

(CD117) which is critical for development and function of ICC. Blockade of c-Kit function resulted in mice lacking ICC in the gastrointestinal wall. With electrophysiological examinations Maeda et al. revealed that the slow wave of the guts peristalsis was missing in the animals affected bowel segments. These findings suggested that ICC and c-Kit play a crucial role in the development of the pacemaker system that is required for the generation of autonomic gut motility. This discovery modified the concept of how gastrointestinal motility is controlled dramatically by suggesting that smooth muscle cells need more than just impulses from enteric nerve cells to generate organized gastrointestinal motility. Meanwhile, it is well established that ICC serve as electrical pacemakers and generate spontaneous electrical slow waves in the gastrointestinal tract (Takaki, 2003; Ward et al., 2004). Slow waves organize gut contractions into phasic contractions that are the basis for peristalsis and segmentation.

3. Physiology and function of ICC

The motility of the gastrointestinal tract drives its contents towards the aboral parts of the gut. Local pendular, non-propulsive mixing and propulsive peristaltic waves are taking part in this process. Still, the control of these movements is poorly understood. The intrinsic enteric nervous system consists of more than 100 million neurons. That is approximately the same amount than can be found in the spinal cord. The enteric nerve system therefore represents a complex integrative system which processes sensoric input and motoric output on a highly sophisticated level. As we know today, the regulation by motor neurotransmission is much more complicated than simple release of transmitter from nerve terminals and binding of receptors on smooth muscle cells.

A central part of the gastrointestinal motility regulation are ICC which are closely connected to smooth muscle cells and enteric neurons by gap junctions. They generate rhythmic pacemaker activity which triggers the slow depolarizing membrane potentials accompanying the contractions in smooth muscle cells. The term "slow waves" was coined because of their low frequency of occurrence and long duration (Mostafa et al., 2010). As recent studies confirm, ICC-MY are the specific pacemaker cells in the gut. Even after blocking the gut's neuronal function completely, recordings from isolated muscle cells show a regular pacemaker pattern generated by ICC. The pacemaker potentials generated by ICC-MY are passively propagated to the smooth muscle cells via gap junctions to generate slow waves (Huang and Xu, 2010). Special ICC subpopulations can transfer pacemaker depolarisation from ICC-MY deep into the distant bundles of circular muscle, orchestrating contractile patterns such as the spreading ring of contraction in peristalsis or the alternating contractions of segmentation (Sanders and Ward, 2007).

Slow wave driven peristalsis varies between the segments of the gastrointestinal tract. Whereas in the stomach a primarily unidirectional peristalsis is present, the colon shows a digestive activity which is much more sensitive to modulation by distension or neuronal input. The exact mechanisms for the generation of pacemaker currents still remain controversial. The activity of a pacemaker channel is required, to initiate the pacemaker current. Many studies have shown that inhibitors of calcium channels like cyclopiazonic acid inhibited slow waves and pacemaker currents in ICC (Ward et al., 2000). Therefore, intracellular calcium seems to play an important role in the pacemaker activities. Meanwhile more and more evidence has been gathered that changes in intracellular calcium levels activate non-selective cation channels and/or calcium-activated chloride channels to conduct the depolarizing pacemaker currents in ICC (Takaki et al., 2010). The frequency of the generated slow wave determines the contractile frequency of the gut.

Additionally to acting as a mere pacemaker for the guts peristalsis, ICC seem to play an important role in transducing inputs from enteric motor neurons. Ultrastructural studies have found synapse-like membrane densities between ICC-IM and enteric nerve terminals. Accessorily, a variety of receptors for neurotransmitters have been identified in ICC. In murine fundus it was shown that ICC-IM were closely associated with cholinergic neurons (Huang and Xu, 2010). These and other results suggest that ICC-IM mediate neurotransmission and signalling between autonomic nerves and smooth muscle cells in the gut (Takaki et al., 2010). Both of the dominant enteric neural motor inputs, i.e. cholinergic and nitrergic, can influence slow wave frequency through communication with ICC (Ward et al., 2004).

The recent data confirms the complexity of gastrointestinal motility and credits ICC with at least three major regulative functions: 1st generating of spontaneous electrical rhythms of the gut known as slow waves, 2nd creating a propagation pathway for slow waves to adjacent parts of the guts musculature, and 3rd mediating excitatory cholinergic and inhibitory nitrergic neuronal inputs from the enteric nervous system. Finally, some novel studies indicate that ICC may serve as nonneural stretch receptors in gut muscle, affecting both smooth muscle excitability and slow wave frequency (Quigley, 2010). Considering the immense effects of ICC on intestinal motility, it should be no surprise that ICC have been in the focus of attention in various gastrointestinal motility disorders. In fact, decreased ICC numbers and abnormal integrity are meanwhile considered a hallmark in diabetic gastropathy as well as in slow transit constipation (Farrugia, 2008). Alterations in the ICC network are thought to have a dramatic effect on the motility of the gastrointestinal system.

4. The role of ICC in gastrointestinal motility disorders

Many gastrointestinal motility disorders have been associated with abnormal numbers or disorders of ICC so far (Burns, 2007; Farrugia, 2008; Ordog et al., 2009). For the clinical workup it is important to keep in mind that no reference values for ICC numbers or network structure have been published. This is due to the different types of biopsy preparations and stainings in use. Therefore, study results have to be interpreted with great care, and comparisons of results from different laboratories can be misleading. For the visualisation of c-Kit (CD117), a receptor tyrosine kinase expressed by ICC, a variety of antibodies is available, yielding results of different quality. Not until 2009 an optimized protocol for improved ICC detection in gastrointestinal motility disorders was presented (Garrity et al., 2009). Since ICC appear very sensitive to hypoxia, abnormalities noted on pathological examination of specimen may also reflect tissue ischemia prior to fixation (Farrugia, 2008).

Most of the ideas regarding the cause of several gastrointestinal motor disorders are still derived from animal models. Because human biopsy samples are still rarely obtained for ICC staining, most case reports published in the literature are describing only a few cases each. However, meanwhile several papers, using a variety of techniques, describing abnormal ICC networks in gastrointestinal motility disorders, have been published. A pubmed search with the keywords "interstitial cells of Cajal" and "gastrointestinal motility" now yields more than 400 results. Whether the observed changes in ICC morphology are primary, secondary or merely epiphenomic remains still much debated (Gladman and

Knowles, 2008). Some authors propose that changes in ICC networks in gastrointestinal diseases are due to inflammatory processes or mechanically induced due to long lasting intestinal obstruction. In a number of human motility disorders with abnormal ICC, however, there is no overt inflammation or dilatation suggesting that this cannot be the only reason for the observed ICC abnormalities (Farrugia, 2008).

4.1 Achalasia

ICC of the intramuscular subtype are found in the muscular layers of the oesophagus and especially in the lower oesophageal sphincter (LES). Ultrastructural damage and loss of ICC-IM in the oesophagus have been reported in achalasia (Faussone-Pellegrini and Cortesini, 1985; Streutker et al., 2007). The disease is characterized by an impaired relaxation of the LES, leading to dilatation of the proximal segments of the oesophagus. Etiologically a loss of inhibitory nerves and progressive degeneration of ganglion cells containing vasoactive intestinal peptide (VIP) and nitric oxide (NO) are suspected to be major causes of LES dysfunction (Negreanu et al., 2008). The pathogenetic role of ICC in achalasia is still much debated. Sanders et al. suggest that loss of ICC in the LES would lead to loss of cholingergic tone and changes in LES tension subsequently (Sanders et al., 2002). Although the close anatomical relationship between ICC and cholinergic neurons is well established in electron microscopy, appropriate studies to determine the functional effect of ICC on the regulation of LES relaxation are still lacking.

4.2 Gastroesophageal reflux disease (GERD)

GERD is one of the most common causes for patients to visit a gastroenterologist. The major mechanism is a transient relaxation of the LES (Kaltenbach et al., 2006). Typical symptoms of heartburn and regurgitation are temporarily encountered by almost 20% of the general adult population. However, no specific histopathological abnormalities of ICC have been found and described so far in humans. Animal studies with ICC lacking W/W^v mice showed a normal swallow induced LES relaxation, contradicting a significant role of ICC in the pathogenesis of reflux disease (Dickens et al., 2001). Secondary changes to the ICC architecture may be induced, when GERD is complicated by severe oesophagitis, oesophageal ulcers or Barret's oesophagus (Negreanu et al., 2008).

4.3 Diabetic gastroenteropathy

Gastroparesis is defined as slow gastric emptying which could not be explained by mechanical obstruction. Up to 30-60% of diabetic patients develop associated symptoms, e.g. dysphagia, heartburn, nausea, abdominal pain, or discomfort. In the long term, gastroparesis may lead to more severe symptoms like nutritional insufficiency, electrolyte imbalance, and impaired glycaemic control (Koch, 1999). The pathomechanisms leading to diabetic gastroparesis are complex and are usually interpreted as a consequence of damage to the autonomic nerve system. Only recently studies addressed the role of ICC loss and dysfunction in the pathophysiology of diabetic gastroenteropathy (Ordog, 2008).

Well characterized animal models have been established for the research of diabetes mellitus type 1. In studies with non-obese diabetic mice (NOD-mice), Ordog et al. showed clearly reduced ICC networks by c-Kit immunofluorescence and electron microscopy in the gastric corpus and antrum in comparison with controls. Both ICC-IM and ICC-MY were affected. Additionally, myenteric ICC were also reduced in the colon. In humans ICC loss in the stomach has also been well documented. In four of nine patients with diabetic gastroparesis profound loss of ICC was observed in biopsy samples of the gastric wall. In another study the same authors reported that nine of 23 patients with gastroparesis showed complete absence of ICC in their antrum biopsies (Forster et al., 2005).

Whether ICC of the small intestine and colon are also affected in humans with diabetes is controversial. Human data is still sparse and patients often suffer from additional maladies such as colonic cancer, which may lead to misinterpretations of the data. In rodent models, however, changes in ICC morphology could also be observed in the proximal and distal colon. However, slow wave frequencies, velocities and extracellular amplitudes were unchanged in a recent study with streptozotocin treated diabetic rats (Lammers et al., 2011), challenging the hypothesis that ICC reduction is severe enough to effect slow wave propagation in the bowel.

Regarding the stomach, the question is, whether the demonstrated changes in ICC morphology are somehow related to the impairment of gastric function in diabetic gastropathy. Delayed emptying of nutrient liquids and solids is caused primarily by antral hypomotility. Reduced smooth muscle contractions as a result of diabetic myopathy and a reduction of pacing electrical slow waves may contribute to the gastric stasis. The role of ICC in the generation and propagation of gastric electrical slow waves is well-established (Ordog, 2008). Abnormal slow wave activity has been shown in different rodent models for diabetes type 1 and 2 combined with diffuse reduction of ICC (Takano et al., 1998). Diabetic rodents showed signs of gastroparesis as well as gastric dysrhythmias. The electrical abnormalities resemble those typically found in human diabetic patients. Thus, reduction in ICC most likely plays a key role in the pathogenesis of diabetic gastroparesis by contributing to gastric hypomotility and delayed gastric emptying.

4.4 Infantile hypertrophic pyloric stenosis

Pyloric stenosis is a congenital disorder characterized by hypertrophy of the inner muscle ring of the pylorus. Signs of delayed gastric emptying are usually not present at birth. Vomiting often starts around the age of three weeks. The etiology is unknown, but abnormal innervation of the pyloric muscle has been implicated. Some studies showed absence of ICC in the hypertrophic circular muscle layer in infants with hypertrophic pyloric stenosis, along with loss of peptidergic and nitric oxide containing nerves (Vanderwinden and Rumessen, 1999). The authors propose the loss of ICC may contribute to the lack of antropyloric coordination and therefore aggravate vomiting and the proper passage of food through the pylorus. An interesting but still unproven theory is that delayed ICC maturation might be one reason explaining the lack of ICC found in immunohistochemnistry and electron microscopy. However, more data is needed to specify the role of ICC in the pathogenesis of hypertrophic pyloric stenosis.

4.5 Slow transit constipation (STC)

Patients suffering from STC show a normal gut diameter and have a prolonged colonic transit. In the majority of cases STC is of unknown etiology. However, it is now well established that ICC play an important role in the pathophysiology of STC. It is plausible that a loss of pacemaker cells would be associated with decrease in colonic transit. Studies proved that ICC density in the colon of patients was significantly decreased compared with those of normal patients (He et al., 2000; Lyford et al., 2002). Expression of *c-kit* mRNA and c-Kit protein in the colon were also decreased in STC, suggesting an important role of the c-Kit signal pathway in the ICC reduction (Tong et al., 2005). Remarkably, these changes in ICC morphology are often accompanied with loss of enteric neurons (Lee et al., 2005) emphasizing the very close relationship between ICC and intrinsic nerves and glial cells. However, a recent study using an automated cellular imaging system for immunohistochemical detection of c-Kit (CD117) showed no significant depletion of ICC. The authors propose that the mere quantification of ICC numbers in the bowel wall may not provide sufficient information on the functional status, since mediation from cholinergic and nitrergic nerves must also be intact for correct ICC function (Toman et al., 2006). Nevertheless, the observed changes in ICC numbers and integrity in patients with STC suggest an important role of ICC when elucidating reduced gastrointestianal motor activity. This has already led some pathology laboratories to include a stain for c-Kit as part of their routine evaluation of specimens resected from patients with STC (Garrity et al., 2009). Future studies will help to understand the exact physiologic and pathopysiologic nature of ICC in STC.

4.6 Chronic intestinal pseudo-obstruction

The term chronic intestinal pseudo-obstruction is used for a group of disorders showing symptoms of intestinal obstruction in the absence of any anatomical or mechanical lesion. Underlying the disease are pathologic disorders from intestinal neuropathy to intestinal myopathy or both. Absence of ICC has been already suggested to be a causative factor leading to intestinal pseudo-obstruction in adults (Vanderwinden and Rumessen, 1999). Yamataka et al. reported abnormal distribution of myenteric ICC in an infant using immunohistochemistry with antihuman c-Kit serum (Yamataka et al., 1998). Recently, one child with total absence of ICC in the myenteric plexus of the distal ileum and colon was reported (Struijs et al., 2008). Feldstein showed altered networks of ICC in a 14-year-old boy (Feldstein et al., 2003). Additionally, delayed maturation of ICC, with normalisation of ICC numbers in subsequent biopsy specimen, has been reported in cases of neonatal pseudo-obstruction (Kenny et al., 1998b).

These findings strongly suggest an important etiologic role for ICC at least in some patients with intestinal pseudo-obstruction. Although many more factors may contribute to manifestation and presentation of the disease, the existent data demonstrates that abnormalities of ICC should be considered early in the diagnostic workup of children with intestinal pseudo-obstruction.

4.7 Congenital aganglionic megacolon (Hirschsprung's disease)

In Hirschsprung's disease the intrinsic enteric nervous system is absent in a segment of the gastrointestinal tract. Mostly found in the distal colon, the aganglionosis may also involve large portions of the entire bowel. Some specimen from the aganglionic region of the colon showed reduced ICC numbers and damaged ICC networks (Wang et al., 2009). Other studies however, point out a high heterogeneity in ICC values within a group of Hirschsprung's patients (Bettolli et al., 2008). Hypothetically, the depletion of ICC in the muscular layer of the gut may contribute to the inability of the smooth muscle to relax. Together with the lack of neurons, a defective initiation of pacemaker currents may also contribute to the motility dysfunction in affected bowel segments. Nevertheless, Hirschsprung's disease remains a heterogenous and multigenetic disease and a routine immunohistochemnistry for ICC seems not helpful in differentiation between the healthy and the aganglionic part of the bowel today. Genetic evidence recently confirmed already the absence of linkage between hereditary forms of Hirschsprung's disease and the region of the ICC-regulating gene *c-kit* (Dow et al., 1994; Mostafa et al., 2010).

4.8 Idiopathic megacolon

In contrast to the congenital megacolon known as Hirschsprung's disease, patients with acquired megacolon show no aganglionic bowel segments and the enteric innervation seems to be intact. Thus, it had been proposed that colonic dysmotility in these patients might as well result from alterations of ICC. Accordingly, some studies of patients with idiopathic megabowel showed decreased ICC density (Lee et al., 2005; Wedel et al., 2002). By contrast, another study of sixty-three patients with megacolon showed no consistent alterations in colonic ICC histology (Meier-Ruge et al., 2006). The results suggest once again that ICC might play an important etiologic role, however more systematic studies are needed to determine the detailed pathomechanisms.

4.9 Children with anorectal malformations

Anorectal malformations comprise a wide spectrum of diseases, which involve the distal anus and rectum as well as the urinary and genital tracts. Defects range from minor anal anomalies to very complex cloacal malformations, which are often associated with other anomalies (Levitt and Pena, 2007). The etiology of such malformations remains unclear and is likely multifactorial. However, in recent years a dramatic progress in operation techniques has improved prognosis significantly.

Constipation, eventually leading to megarectum and functional outlet obstruction, is a common postsurgical problem faced by more than a half of all patients with anorectal malformations. Although in some of these patients aganglionosis or neuronal intestinal dysplasia have been reported, no plausible theory could explain colonic hypomotility satisfactorily so far. Often these symptoms have been attributed to associated abnormalities of the sacral roots or to inherent abnormalities of the myenteric plexus.

Using monoclonal mouse antibody against c-Kit, Kenny et al. reported marked abnormalities in density and distribution of c-Kit-positive ICC in the sigmoid colon in 7 of 12 patients with high or intermediate anorectal malformations (Kenny et al., 1998a). Since no electron microscopy was applied, the authors state that it is uncertain, if the loss of c-Kit immunoreactivity was caused by phenotypic loss of c-Kit antigen, or by complete absence of ICC. The latter would advance speculations that genes involved in gut segmentation and hindgut differentiation are also essential for ICC development. Supporting this, a lower density of ICC in the terminal intestine was recently observed in rats with ethylenethiourea-induced anorectal malformations (Macedo et al., 2008). Although not enough sufficient data is available today, congenital defects in interstitial pacemaker cells may, additionally to other factors, contribute to the colonic hypomobility in patients with anorectal malformations.

4.10 Patients with mutations of *c-kit* and constipation

Signals through the c-Kit receptor tyrosine kinase are essential for development and differentiation of erythrocytes, melanocytes, germ cells, mast cells, and ICC. Gain-of-function mutations of *c-kit* result in the development of mast cell and germ cell tumors, and of ICC tumors called gastrointestinal stromal tumors (GIST), respectively (Kitamura and Hirotab, 2004). In mice the W locus was demonstrated to encode c-Kit, and meanwhile various types of mutants have been reported. Animal models with loss-of-function mutations in the *c-kit* gene compromise the regular development of ICC in the gut (Alberti et al., 2007; Maeda et al., 1992; Sanders and Ward, 2007). In humans however, no homozygote loss-of-function mutations have been reported so far.

Recently one juvenile patient was described whose biopsy specimen showed only few ICC in the ileum and complete absence of ICC in the colon (Breuer et al., 2010). The mutational analysis of Kit in this patient revealed multiple genetic alterations at the level of mRNA which potentially could result in a loss of function of the Kit protein. According to this, it was suggested that the genetic alterations of *c-kit* might lead to alterations in ICC architecture and function.

By now animal studies have already shown that point mutations in the proto-oncogene *c-kit* correlate with abnormal intestinal contractions *in vitro* (Isozaki et al., 1995). Kit mutations might therefore explain cases of patients with megacolon or small transit constipation who show histopathological defects or depletion of ICC. The W^{sh}/W^{sh} c-Kit mutant illustrates the complexity of Kit-regulated ICC differentiation. Although leading to a general absence of ICC in the intestine due to an inversion mutation upstream the promoter region, a subpopulation of special ICC in the deep muscular plexuses (ICC-DMP) developed normally in mutant mice. These findings suggest that ICC-DMP may develop and differentiate without c-Kit expression (Iino et al., 2009).

5. Summary

Constipation and fecal impaction are frequent and distressing complaints in gastroenterology. In most cases a sufficient treatment including changes in lifestyle, activity, and food, with the additional use of laxatives is possible. However, the treatment of severe forms of constipation may constitute a difficult task.

In recent years the role of ICC in gastrointestinal motility is increasingly recognized. Throughout the whole gastrointestinal tract ICC-MY and ICC-IM coordinate smooth muscle activity and guarantee the physiologic course of peristalsis. Whereas ICC-MY act as pacemaker cells to generate slow waves driven by changes of voltage dependent calcium channels, ICC-IM mediate neurotransmission between enteric neurons and smooth muscle cells. Meanwhile lots of cases with histological alterations in ICC morphology have been presented in patients with different types of constipation. However, it occasionally remains unclear, whether morphological alterations of ICC are based on congenital developmental anomalies or whether they are a consequence of long term constipation with secondary damage of the guts neuroarchitecture. Nevertheless, the new insights in ICC physiology and function present a new aspect for gastroenterologists to focus on, when dealing with patients suffering from severe forms of constipation. Clinicians should consider involvement of ICC early in the diagnostic process of motility disorders. Further investigations may lead to the routine staining and evaluation of ICC-morphology in intestinal biopsy specimen.

Although the knowledge of the role of ICC in gastrointestinal disorders is increasing rapidly, no major progress has been achieved in treatment so far. The Kit inhibitor Imatinib mesylate has been shown to be effective in Kit expressing tumors (GISTs), but no drugs improving loss of c-Kit function are available today. Eventually new medications modulating gastrointestinal peristalsis may be provided in the future. Replacement of defective pacemaker cells however, will be a prospective promise of genetic therapy at best.

6. References

Alberti, E., Mikkelsen, H. B., Wang, X. Y., Diaz, M., Larsen, J. O., Huizinga, J. D., and Jimenez, M. (2007). Pacemaker activity and inhibitory neurotransmission in the colon of Ws/Ws mutant rats. Am J Physiol Gastrointest Liver Physiol *292*, G1499-1510.

Bettolli, M., De Carli, C., Jolin-Dahel, K., Bailey, K., Khan, H. F., Sweeney, B., Krantis, A., Staines, W. A., and Rubin, S. (2008). Colonic dysmotility in postsurgical patients with Hirschsprung's disease. Potential significance of abnormalities in the interstitial cells of Cajal and the enteric nervous system. J Pediatr Surg *43*, 1433-1438.

Breuer, C., Oh, J., Molderings, G. J., Schemann, M., Kuch, B., Mayatepek, E., and Adam, R. (2010). Therapy-refractory gastrointestinal motility disorder in a child with c-kit mutations. World J Gastroenterol *16*, 4363-4366.

Burns, A. J. (2007). Disorders of interstitial cells of Cajal. J Pediatr Gastroenterol Nutr *45 Suppl 2*, S103-106.

Cajal, S. R. (1893). Sur les ganglions et plexus nerveux d'intestin. C R Roc Biol Paris *5*, 217-223.

Cajal, S. R. (1911). Histology of the nervous system of man and vertebrates. translation by Swanson and Swanson, Oxford University Press 1995, 891-942.

Dickens, E. J., Edwards, F. R., and Hirst, G. D. (2001). Selective knockout of intramuscular interstitial cells reveals their role in the generation of slow waves in mouse stomach. J Physiol *531*, 827-833.

Dow, E., Cross, S., Wolgemuth, D. J., Lyonnet, S., Mulligan, L. M., Mascari, M., Ladda, R., and Williamson, R. (1994). Second locus for Hirschsprung disease/Waardenburg syndrome in a large Mennonite kindred. Am J Med Genet *53*, 75-80.

Farrugia, G. (2008). Interstitial cells of Cajal in health and disease. Neurogastroenterol Motil *20 Suppl 1*, 54-63.

Faussone-Pellegrini, M. S., and Cortesini, C. (1985). The muscle coat of the lower esophageal sphincter in patients with achalasia and hypertensive sphincter. An electron microscopic study. J Submicrosc Cytol *17*, 673-685.

Faussone-Pellegrini, M. S., and Thuneberg, L. (1999). Guide to the identification of interstitial cells of Cajal. Microsc Res Tech *47*, 248-266.

Feldstein, A. E., Miller, S. M., El-Youssef, M., Rodeberg, D., Lindor, N. M., Burgart, L. J., Szurszewski, J. H., and Farrugia, G. (2003). Chronic intestinal pseudoobstruction associated with altered interstitial cells of cajal networks. J Pediatr Gastroenterol Nutr *36*, 492-497.

Forster, J., Damjanov, I., Lin, Z., Sarosiek, I., Wetzel, P., and McCallum, R. W. (2005). Absence of the interstitial cells of Cajal in patients with gastroparesis and correlation with clinical findings. J Gastrointest Surg *9*, 102-108.

Garrity, M. M., Gibbons, S. J., Smyrk, T. C., Vanderwinden, J. M., Gomez-Pinilla, P. J., Nehra, A., Borg, M., and Farrugia, G. (2009). Diagnostic challenges of motility disorders: optimal detection of CD117+ interstitial cells of Cajal. Histopathology *54*, 286-294.

Gladman, M. A., and Knowles, C. H. (2008). Novel concepts in the diagnosis, pathophysiology and management of idiopathic megabowel. Colorectal Dis *10*, 531-538; discussion 538-540.

He, C. L., Burgart, L., Wang, L., Pemberton, J., Young-Fadok, T., Szurszewski, J., and Farrugia, G. (2000). Decreased interstitial cell of cajal volume in patients with slow-transit constipation. Gastroenterology *118*, 14-21.

Huang, X., and Xu, W. X. (2010). The pacemaker functions of visceral interstitial cells of Cajal. Sheng Li Xue Bao *62*, 387-397.

Iino, S., Horiguchi, K., and Nojyo, Y. (2009). W(sh)/W(sh) c-Kit mutant mice possess interstitial cells of Cajal in the deep muscular plexus layer of the small intestine. Neurosci Lett *459*, 123-126.

Isozaki, K., Hirota, S., Nakama, A., Miyagawa, J., Shinomura, Y., Xu, Z., Nomura, S., and Kitamura, Y. (1995). Disturbed intestinal movement, bile reflux to the stomach, and deficiency of c-kit-expressing cells in Ws/Ws mutant rats. Gastroenterology *109*, 456-464.

Kaltenbach, T., Crockett, S., and Gerson, L. B. (2006). Are lifestyle measures effective in patients with gastroesophageal reflux disease? An evidence-based approach. Arch Intern Med *166*, 965-971.

Kenny, S. E., Connell, M. G., Rintala, R. J., Vaillant, C., Edgar, D. H., and Lloyd, D. A. (1998a). Abnormal colonic interstitial cells of Cajal in children with anorectal malformations. J Pediatr Surg *33*, 130-132.

Kenny, S. E., Vanderwinden, J. M., Rintala, R. J., Connell, M. G., Lloyd, D. A., Vanderhaegen, J. J., and De Laet, M. H. (1998b). Delayed maturation of the interstitial cells of Cajal: a new diagnosis for transient neonatal pseudoobstruction. Report of two cases. J Pediatr Surg *33*, 94-98.

Kitamura, Y., and Hirotab, S. (2004). Kit as a human oncogenic tyrosine kinase. Cell Mol Life Sci *61*, 2924-2931.

Koch, K. L. (1999). Diabetic gastropathy: gastric neuromuscular dysfunction in diabetes mellitus: a review of symptoms, pathophysiology, and treatment. Dig Dis Sci *44*, 1061-1075.

Lammers, W. J., Al-Bloushi, H. M., Al-Eisae, S. A., Al-Dhaheri, F. A., Stephen, B. S., John, R., Dhanasekaran, S., and Karam, S. M. (2011). Slow wave propagation and ICC plasticity in the small intestine of diabetic rats. Exp Physiol.

Lee, J. I., Park, H., Kamm, M. A., and Talbot, I. C. (2005). Decreased density of interstitial cells of Cajal and neuronal cells in patients with slow-transit constipation and acquired megacolon. J Gastroenterol Hepatol *20*, 1292-1298.

Levitt, M. A., and Pena, A. (2007). Anorectal malformations. Orphanet J Rare Dis *2*, 33.

Lyford, G. L., He, C. L., Soffer, E., Hull, T. L., Strong, S. A., Senagore, A. J., Burgart, L. J., Young-Fadok, T., Szurszewski, J. H., and Farrugia, G. (2002). Pan-colonic decrease in interstitial cells of Cajal in patients with slow transit constipation. Gut *51*, 496-501.

Macedo, M., Martins, J. L., Meyer, K. F., and Soares, I. C. (2008). Study of density of interstitial cells of cajal in the terminal intestine of rats with anorectal malformation. Eur J Pediatr Surg *18*, 75-79.

Maeda, H., Yamagata, A., Nishikawa, S., Yoshinaga, K., Kobayashi, S., Nishi, K., and Nishikawa, S. (1992). Requirement of c-kit for development of intestinal pacemaker system. Development *116*, 369-375.

Meier-Ruge, W. A., Muller-Lobeck, H., Stoss, F., and Bruder, E. (2006). The pathogenesis of idiopathic megacolon. Eur J Gastroenterol Hepatol *18*, 1209-1215.

Mostafa, R. M., Moustafa, Y. M., and Hamdy, H. (2010). Interstitial cells of Cajal, the Maestro in health and disease. World J Gastroenterol *16*, 3239-3248.

Negreanu, L. M., Assor, P., Mateescu, B., and Cirstoiu, C. (2008). Interstitial cells of Cajal in the gut--a gastroenterologist's point of view. World J Gastroenterol *14*, 6285-6288.

Ordog, T. (2008). Interstitial cells of Cajal in diabetic gastroenteropathy. Neurogastroenterol Motil *20*, 8-18.

Ordog, T., Hayashi, Y., and Gibbons, S. J. (2009). Cellular pathogenesis of diabetic gastroenteropathy. Minerva Gastroenterol Dietol *55*, 315-343.

Quigley, E. M. (2010). What we have learned about colonic motility: normal and disturbed. Curr Opin Gastroenterol *26*, 53-60.

Sanders, K. M., and Ward, S. M. (2007). Kit mutants and gastrointestinal physiology. J Physiol *578*, 33-42.

Sanders, K. M., Ward, S. M., and Daniel, E. E. (2002). ICC in neurotransmission: hard to swallow a lack of involvement. Gastroenterology *122*, 1185-1186; author reply 1186-1187.

Streutker, C. J., Huizinga, J. D., Driman, D. K., and Riddell, R. H. (2007). Interstitial cells of Cajal in health and disease. Part I: normal ICC structure and function with associated motility disorders. Histopathology *50*, 176-189.

Struijs, M. C., Diamond, I. R., Pencharz, P. B., Chang, K. T., Viero, S., Langer, J. C., and Wales, P. W. (2008). Absence of the interstitial cells of Cajal in a child with chronic pseudoobstruction. J Pediatr Surg *43*, e25-29.

Takaki, M. (2003). Gut pacemaker cells: the interstitial cells of Cajal (ICC). J Smooth Muscle Res *39*, 137-161.

Takaki, M., Suzuki, H., and Nakayama, S. (2010). Recent advances in studies of spontaneous activity in smooth muscle: ubiquitous pacemaker cells. Prog Biophys Mol Biol *102*, 129-135.

Takano, H., Imaeda, K., Koshita, M., Xue, L., Nakamura, H., Kawase, Y., Hori, S., Ishigami, T., Kurono, Y., and Suzuki, H. (1998). Alteration of the properties of gastric smooth muscle in the genetically hyperglycemic OLETF rat. J Auton Nerv Syst *70*, 180-188.

Toman, J., Turina, M., Ray, M., Petras, R. E., Stromberg, A. J., and Galandiuk, S. (2006). Slow transit colon constipation is not related to the number of interstitial cells of Cajal. Int J Colorectal Dis *21*, 527-532.

Tong, W. D., Liu, B. H., Zhang, L. Y., Xiong, R. P., Liu, P., and Zhang, S. B. (2005). Expression of c-kit messenger ribonucleic acid and c-kit protein in sigmoid colon of patients with slow transit constipation. Int J Colorectal Dis *20*, 363-367.

Vanderwinden, J. M., and Rumessen, J. J. (1999). Interstitial cells of Cajal in human gut and gastrointestinal disease. Microsc Res Tech *47*, 344-360.

Wang, H., Zhang, Y., Liu, W., Wu, R., Chen, X., Gu, L., Wei, B., and Gao, Y. (2009). Interstitial cells of Cajal reduce in number in recto-sigmoid Hirschsprung's disease and total colonic aganglionosis. Neurosci Lett *451*, 208-211.

Ward, S. M., Ordog, T., Koh, S. D., Baker, S. A., Jun, J. Y., Amberg, G., Monaghan, K., and Sanders, K. M. (2000). Pacemaking in interstitial cells of Cajal depends upon calcium handling by endoplasmic reticulum and mitochondria. J Physiol *525 Pt 2*, 355-361.

Ward, S. M., Sanders, K. M., and Hirst, G. D. (2004). Role of interstitial cells of Cajal in neural control of gastrointestinal smooth muscles. Neurogastroenterol Motil *16 Suppl 1*, 112-117.

Wedel, T., Spiegler, J., Soellner, S., Roblick, U. J., Schiedeck, T. H., Bruch, H. P., and Krammer, H. J. (2002). Enteric nerves and interstitial cells of Cajal are altered in patients with slow-transit constipation and megacolon. Gastroenterology *123*, 1459-1467.

Yamataka, A., Ohshiro, K., Kobayashi, H., Lane, G. J., Yamataka, T., Fujiwara, T., Sunagawa, M., and Miyano, T. (1998). Abnormal distribution of intestinal pacemaker (C-KIT-positive) cells in an infant with chronic idiopathic intestinal pseudoobstruction. J Pediatr Surg *33*, 859-862.

Skipping Breakfast is Associated with Constipation in Post-Adolescent Female College Students in Japan

Tomoko Fujiwara
Faculty of Home Economics, Ashiya College, Ashiya, Japan

1. Introduction

Intake of food is one of the most effective stimulations that induce bowel movement. Food intake stimulates bowel peristalsis mainly through automatic nerve system (Nobel et al., 2009). On the other hand, it is widely accepted that physiological and/or psychological stresses can induce constipation in women by suppressing the function of parasympathetic nerve networks (Whitehead, 1996).

In general, the dominance of the parasympathetic nerve system while sleeping promotes digestive and absorptive function. In this regard, the time dinner is eaten may be a factor that influences the conditions of bowel movement the following day. In addition, intake of breakfast is an important event that gives an opportunity to empty the bowels in the morning when the work day usually starts (Cummings JH). Accordingly, it is speculated that late intake of dinner or skipping breakfast can disrupt the rhythms of bowel movement, inducing various problems such as constipation.

To support the above speculation, Kunimoto *et al.* reported that skipping breakfast is strongly related to constipation in Japanese working women and signs of this relationship have already appeared in adolescents (Kunimoto *et al.*, 1998). In accordance with this study, we also observed the positive relationship between breakfast skipping and constipation in Japanese young female students (Fujiwara and Nakata, 2010).

In this study, we re-evaluated the relationship between skipping breakfast and bowel movement by conducting an 11-year questionnaire survey (from 2000 to 2010) of 1,877 female college students aged between 18 and 20 years old. We further examined the relationship between dinner time and bowel movement by conducting a single year questionnaire survey in 2010.

2. Methods

2.1 Respondents to a questionnaire

The subjects were yong Japanese women aged from 18 to 20 years old who studied at the Faculty of Home Economics of Ashiya College and Kyoto Bunkyo Junior College. The study protocol was approved by the Committee on Food Culture at Ashiya College. We sent questionnaires to all students who belonged to the Faculty of Home Economics and Child Education between 2000 and 2010. Information regarding the aim of this study was sent with the questionnaire, and consent was obtained from all participants. The total number of the participants in the sequential studies was 1898 and we obtained responses that were suitable for statistical analysis from 1,877 students in the sequential study.

2.2 Questionnaire items

2.2.1 Skipping breakfast

All study participants completed a food-frequency questionnaire about breakfast (food intake until 9:00 am) and were divided into three groups as follows: Group I, having breakfast every morning; Group II, having breakfast one to six times a week; and Group III, having breakfast less than once a week.

2.2.2 Body mass index (BMI) assessment

Information on body mass (kilograms) and height (meters) of all participants were obtained from a physical examination organized by the Health Center at Ashiya College and Kyoto Bunkyo Junior College. BMI was calculated using the formula: body weight in kilograms divided by height in meters squared.

2.2.3 Bowel movement

The frequency of bowel movement was classified into Grade 1 (no more than once a week), Grade 2 (2-6 times a week), and Grade 3 (every day).

2.2.4 Time of dinner intake

Participants in 2010 were divided into three groups according to the time of dinner as follows: Group A, having dinner before 19:00; Group B, having dinner between 19:00 and 21:00; Group C, having dinner after 21:00.

2.3 Statistical analysis

The data are shown as mean ± standard deviation (SD). Differences in the bowel movement among Groups I-III and A-C were analyzed by the Kruskal-Wallis test, followed by the Mann-Whitney test for multiple comparisons. The relationship between BMI and skipping breakfast was analyzed by one-way analysis of variance, followed by Scheffe's F test for multiple comparisons. *P*-values less than 0.05 were considered significant.

3. Results

3.1 Changes over time in the proportions of the population showing various breakfast habits

Among the participants, 1877 students were classified in Groups I, II and III. Annual population rates for breakfast habits between 2000 and 2010 are shown in Figure 1. Population of breakfast skipping has been within 5-22% throughout the study.

3.2 Changes over time in bowel movement scores

There was a tendency for bowel movement scores in Group I to be higher than those in the other groups throughout the study (Figure 1).

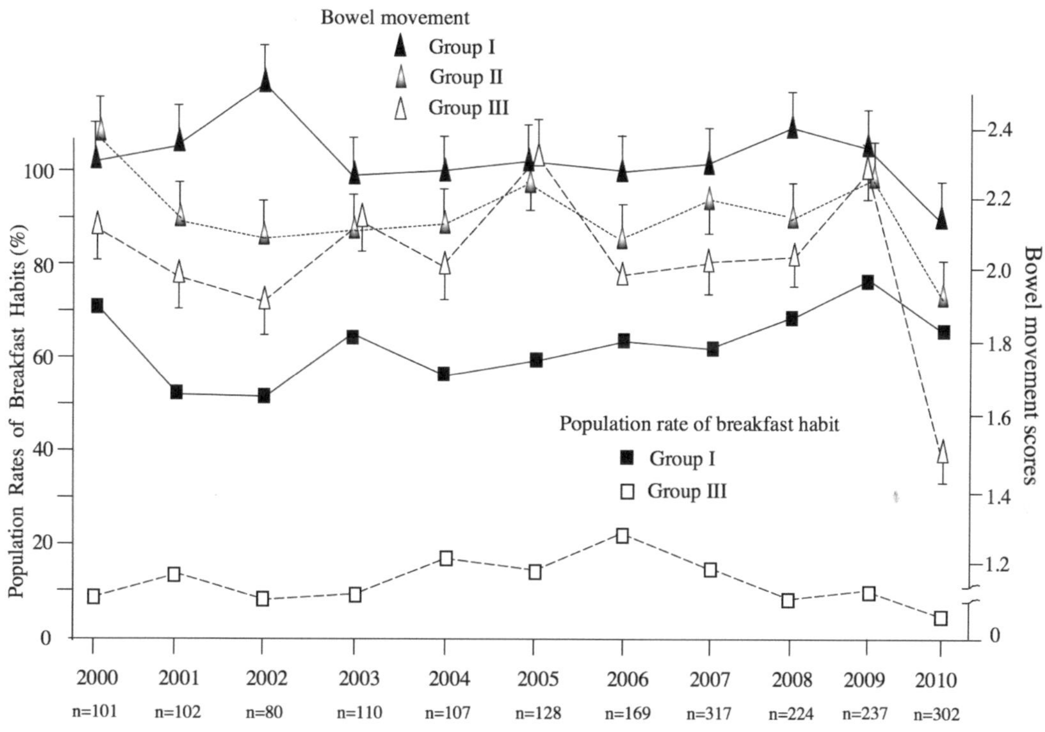

Fig. 1. Changes in population rates and bowel movement scores in Groups I, II and III throughout an 11-year surveillance period from 2000 to 2010. Population of breakfast skipping has been within 5-22% and bowel movement scores in Group I are higher than those in the other groups throughout the study.

3.3 Relationship between breakfast habits and bowel movement scores

The bowel movement score was significantly lower in Group III than in Group I and II (Figure 2).

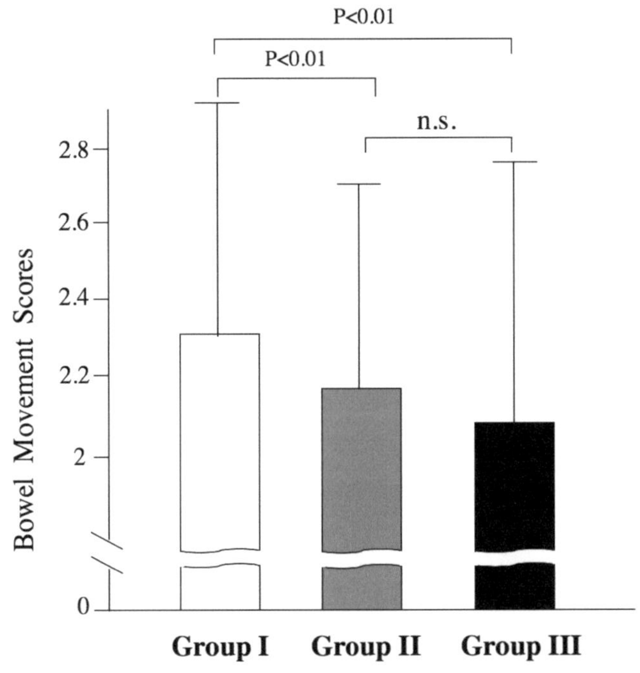

Fig. 2. Relationship between skipping breakfast and bowel movement scores. The bowel movement score was significantly lower in Group III than in Group I and Group II, suggesting that skipping breakfast induced constipation in young students.

3.4 The differences in BMI scores

As shown in Figure 3, there were no significant differences in BMI scores among Group I, II and III. There were no significant changes in BMI scores throughout the observation periods.

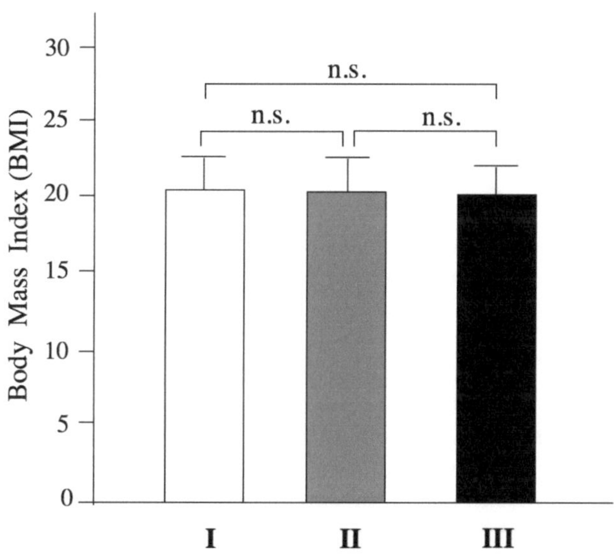

Fig. 3. Relationship between skipping breakfast and BMI. There were no significant changes in BMI scores among three groups.

3.5 Relationship between dinner time and bowel movement scores

Bowel movement scores in Group A were significantly higher than those of the other two groups (Figure 4).

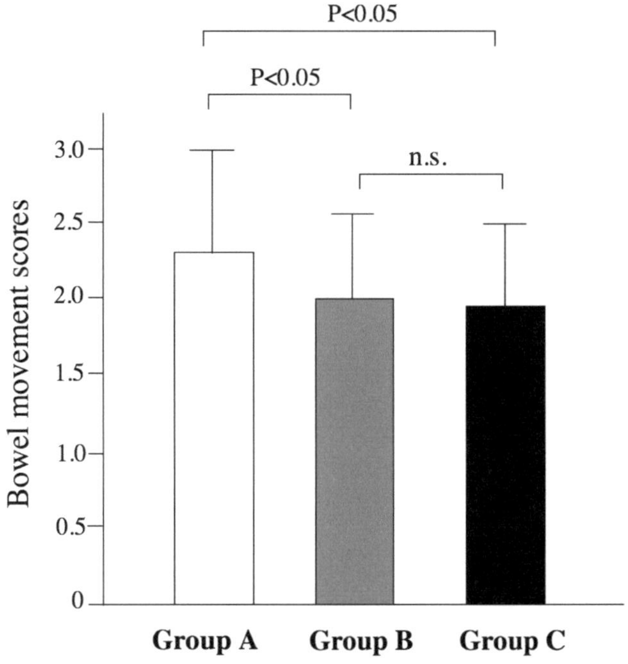

Fig. 4. Relationship between dinner time and bowel movement scores. Bowel movement scores in Group A were significantly higher than those of the other two groups.

4. Discussion

For more than a decade, we have been studying the relationship between food habits and quality of life (QOL) in young Japanese women by analyzing the responses to a questionnaire completed by Ashiya College and Kyoto Bunkyo Junior College students. Since the educational and social environment of these populations remained stable throughout this longitudinal survey, we think that the results obtained from these data convincingly represent annual changes in the status of young Japanese women and provide important information.

We previously reported that skipping breakfast is significantly related with poor physical conditions in Japanese female young students (Fujiwara and Nakata, 2010). The present study showed that small population of young students habitually skipped breakfast. Fortunately, this percentage seems to have decreased in recent years (Figure 1). However, it should be noted that accumulating evidence has been suggesting that habits of food intake considerably affects QOL in women. To support this concern, this study clearly showed that students who skip breakfast have a significantly lower frequency of bowel movement compared with that in young women who eat breakfast (Figure 2). This suggests that skipping breakfast induces constipation in young female students.

In general, food intake especially just after waking up effectively stimulates stomach and induces bowel movement via the parasympathetic nerve pathway. Therefore, it is reasonably speculated that skipping breakfast decreased stimulation to digestive organs in the morning, causing reduction and irregularity of bowel movement. Abnormality in food intake can induce some degree of nutritional defect. Since social activity is relatively high in the morning, skipping breakfast may contribute to a nutritional defect that can affect QOL. However, this study showed that there was no significant difference in BMI among 3 groups (Figure 3). These findings suggest that breakfast skipping had little effects on the total supply of energy for young students and suggested that the positive relationship between breakfast skipping and constipation is due to the disarrangement of the rhythms of automatic nerve systems.

Interestingly, the preliminary study suggested a new proposal that early intake of dinner can improve bowel movement in young female students. Although we cannot exclude the effects of factors accompanying the early intake of dinner, these data notably demonstrated that intake of dinner before 19:00, but not between 19:00 and 21:00, had significant effects on improvement of bowel movement. Considering that intake of dinner between 19:00 and 21:00 has become a common life style practice in modern civilized countries, it is suggested that an intrinsic ideal dietary rhythm for bowel movement in humans differs from our dietary habits.

From the sequential survey conducted in this study, we also found that skipping breakfast is associated with female reproductive disorders such as dysmenorrhea (Fujiwara T, 2003) and proposed that impairment of reproductive function by skipping breakfast may become a trigger for the subsequent onset of gynecologic diseases such as endometriosis in the future (Fujiwara T, 2007). Thus, although the precise mechanisms are still unknown, it is speculated that physiological or pathological conditions of the pelvic organs can be influenced by dietary habits (Fujiwara et al., 2009). Consequently, considering the possibility that constipation influences the environment of pelvic cavity, the relationship between constipation and female genital organic disorders should be examined in the future.

5. Conclusion

In conclusion, by conducting a questionnaire survey, this study suggested that early intake of dinner promoted, while skipping breakfast reduced bowel movement in young Japanese female students. These findings support the current concept that dietary habits regulate bowel functions. Since constipation can cause psychological and/or organic disorders, this issue should be re-evaluated from the perspective of dietary rhythm.

6. References

Cummings, J.H. (1984) Constipation, dietary fibre and the control of large bowel function. *Postgraduate Medical Journal*, 60, 811-819.

Fujiwara, T. (2003). Skipping breakfast is associated with dysmenorrhea in young women in Japan. *International Journal of Food Science and Nutrition*, 54, 505-509.

Fujiwara, T. (2007). Diet during adolescence is a trigger for subsequent development of dysmenorrhea in young women. *International Journal of Food Science and Nutrition,* 58, 437-444.

Fujiwara, T., Sato, N., Awaji, H., Sakamoto, H., & Nakata, R. (2009). Skipping Breakfast Adversely Affects Menstrual Disorders in Young College Students. *International Journal of Food Science and Nutrition,* 26, 1-9.

Fujiwara, T. & Nakata R. (2010) Skipping breakfast is associated with reproductive dysfunction in post-adolescent female college students. *Appetite,* 55, 714-717.

Kunimoto, M., Nishi, M., & Sasaki K. (1998) The relation between irregular bowel movement and the lifestyle of working women. *Hepatogastroenterology,* 45, 956-960.

Noble, E.J., Harris, R., Hosie, K.B., Thomas, S. & Lewis, S.J. (2009) Gum chewing reduces postoperative ileus? A systematic review and meta-analysis. *International Journal of Surgery,* 7, 100-105.

Whitehead, W.E. (1996) Psychosocial aspects of functional gastrointestinal disorders. *Gastroenterology Clinics of North America,* 25, 21-34.

5

Irritable Bowel Syndrome and Constipation

Brian C. Dobson
Performance Edge Systems
New Zealand

1. Introduction

A hypothetical model of the digestive system that can create the symptoms of Irritable Bowel Syndrome (IBS) was originally published as (Dobson, 2008). This chapter presents the model and includes additional research. The model accounts for all types of IBS.

A mechanism that creates **constipation**, improved diagnostic criteria, suggestions for testing the model, treatment options, diagrams showing how the autonomic nervous system creates IBS symptoms, and photomicrographs of the insoluble food fibres triggering IBS, are included.

The data necessary to write this chapter was collected over four decades. Initially the aim of the research was to treat a member of the author's family who has severe IBS-D, and successful treatment programs have been developed. In addition the observed symptoms of all types of IBS, have suggested the hypothesis on which this chapter is based.

2. A worldwide digestive illness

IBS is one of the most common maladies that a GP encounters. The symptoms of IBS range from mild and intermittent, to severe, continuous and incapacitating. Rates of occurrence have been measured at up to 25% in some countries. The economic burden is tens of billions of dollars annually for the USA alone (Schwetz & Chang, 2004) (Drossman, 2007).

GPs diagnose IBS by eliminating other digestive disorders. The symptoms demonstrate that something is wrong but they can find no visible damage. The GP has few treatment options available and they are often ineffective. The patient goes away and tries to cope. Their days can be miserable. They may suffer from **constipation**, bloating, cramping, diarrhoea, all four, or even none of these and instead, a host of other ailments. They may be unable to work, afraid to eat, and suffer from weight loss & malnutrition. They may have herb & fibre supplements, laxatives, and/or anti-diarrhoea medicines at hand. The author has also noted secondary symptoms such as depression, headache, hallucinations, guts ache, lack of energy, weight loss, skin infections, back pain, aching limbs, athlete's foot, ingrown nails, and other minor problems caused by malnutrition.

2.1 Types of IBS

These three types are widely recognized (Drossman 2007): IBS-C (**constipation** predominant), IBS-D (diarrhoea predominant), and IBS-A or IBS-M (alternating or mixed, **constipation** & diarrhoea).

These descriptions contain the symptoms as observed by the author...

1. IBS-C... the primary symptom is **constipation**. Bloating may be hard to detect but is always present. It begins in the morning when breakfast is eaten and then may disappear overnight. Bowel movements are hard to pass, and diarrhoea never occurs. Borborygmi (gurgling), cramping, and difficulty with fat digestion may be present.
2. IBS-D... the primary symptom is diarrhoea. This usually occurs on arising as the 'morning rush', but it can also happen at other times. When **constipation** is a symptom, bloating is never present. Borborygmi and irritation around the anus are always present. Cramping and difficulty with fat digestion may be present.
3. IBS-A or IBS-M... bloating, **constipation** and diarrhoea that alternate irregularly are the primary symptoms. Borborygmi, irritation around the anus, cramping, and difficulty with fat digestion may be present.

3. The hypothesis

Digestion in the small intestine is a batch process with three sequential sections corresponding to the natural divisions of the intestine. These are the duodenum, the jejunum, and the ileum. It is governed by a brain controller divided into four sub-controllers, each of which has a unique neurotransmitter. Control faults in this process cause the disorder irritable bowel syndrome.

This hypothesis has been created by the author in order to explain the symptoms of IBS that he has observed over a period of decades. It accurately creates all types of IBS when faults occur in its control mechanisms.

3.1 Transport controllers

There are two transport control systems for the process...

1. The primary control system is a brain controller that is part of the autonomic nervous system. It is divided into four sub-controllers. The duodenum, the jejunum & the ileum each have a dedicated transport sub-controller. These three sub-controllers produce output only when input is received. They obtain input from sensors in the walls of the intestine that detect food soup. Output regulates transport and mixing in the small intestine. Correct control happens regardless of the variable input caused by different foods. The food soup is moved backwards and forwards so that chemicals can be mixed in, and the rate of absorption of nutrients & chemicals controlled. It is then transferred to the next section at the correct time, and at the correct speed (slow).
2. A secondary control system called the MMC is applied when primary controller outputs are absent. This is a reflex action of the enteric nervous system. It is normally only active when the intestine has no food in it. When food is present, and the primary controller is defective, the transport speed set by the secondary controller is dependent on the type of foods eaten and the state of the autonomic nervous system. There is no control of mixing or timing, and movement is in the forward direction only. When the speed is too fast, IBS occurs.

3.2 Chemical controllers

Two systems control addition of digestive chemicals to the duodenum...

1. The primary system is the fourth sub-division of the small intestine brain controller. Cells in the wall of the duodenum release CCK hormone (Rehfeld J.F., 2004) into the bloodstream when food soup containing fat is pumped in from the stomach. The brain detects this hormone and sends a nerve signal to the muscle that empties the gall bladder and pancreas. The pancreas provides protease enzymes, lipase enzymes, & bicarbonate. The gall bladder provides bile salts. If this controller is defective, then insufficient chemicals are added to the duodenum.
2. The secondary controller is the enteric nervous system which adds chemicals when it detects; the amount and type of fibre eaten, cooked proteins (meats, fish, & eggs), fruit acids (alpha hydroxy acids), dairy proteins, and some herbs & spices (e.g. ginger). The amount added however is insufficient, and extra must be provided by the primary controller in order to complete the digestive process.

3.3 Primary control faults

The following defects may occur…

1. One or more of the four neurotransmitters in the primary controller may be deficient or absent. This reduces or eliminates output from one or more sub-controllers of the primary controller.
2. A toxic insult may destroy intestinal sensors that provide input to the primary controller. This reduces or eliminates output from the sub-controller of the affected part of the intestine.
3. Surgical procedures may sever input nerves to the primary controller or output nerves from the primary controller to the intestine.
4. Misalignment of neck vertebrae may put pressure on nerves connecting the primary controller to the small intestine.
5. In infancy, development of nerve connections from the brain to the small intestine, may fail to be completed.
6. Any other fault that interrupts communication between the small intestine and the brain.

3.4 IBS-B – Bile deficient IBS

When the neurotransmitter in the primary chemical controller is missing or deficient, insufficient lipases and bile salts are added to the food soup. Undigested fats impair nutrient uptake in the jejunum, and the reabsorbtion of chemicals in the ileum. Indigestion is followed by fast, loose, grey bowel movements containing fat (steatorrhea). The absence of the brown bile pigment stercobilin causes the grey colour, and when fat is present in the colon, the enteric nervous system automatically evacuates it. IBS-B may occur alone but often it accompanies one of the other three types of IBS. When it does, the symptoms of the other types become severe.

3.5 Constipation – Creation of the IBS barrier

The IBS Barrier is created when food soup is present in the small intestine, and a section under the control of the secondary transport controller precedes a section under the control of the primary transport controller. When the primary controller detects the too fast movement of food soup, it constricts the intestine to stop the flow. It will not allow food soup to travel too fast. The Barrier causes the IBS symptoms of bloating and **constipation**.

The Barrier is created by parts of the autonomic nervous system. Variation in the level of activity in this system causes Barrier strength to vary. It is strong on arising when adrenal hormones are released to start the metabolism. The symptoms of the Barrier start when breakfast is eaten. When stress releases more adrenal hormones during the day it again increases in strength. It will relax overnight if adrenal hormones and the autonomic nervous system return to a low level.

3.5.1 IBS-C caused by a neurotransmitter deficiency

There are six forms;

a. The duodenum controller output is deficient or missing. This causes a Barrier to form at the start of the jejunum. When a breakfast containing cereal is eaten, immediate, severe bloating occurs. Backpressure in the duodenum keeps the valve from the gall bladder and pancreas closed, so that insufficient chemicals are added to the food soup (see Diagram 1).
b. Form (a) as above together with IBS-B.
c. The jejunum controller output is deficient or missing. This causes a Barrier to form at the start of the ileum. When a breakfast containing cereal is eaten, borborygmi occurs followed by hard to detect, slight to moderate bloating. Onset of these symptoms is delayed by a few minutes (see Diagram 2).

	Primary controller				
#	Chemical	Duodenum	Jejunum	Ileum	Symptoms
(a)	O	X	O	O	Immediate severe bloating that disappears overnight. Cramping possible. **Constipation**. Steatorrhea. No borborygmi.
(b)	X	X	O	O	Immediate severe bloating that disappears overnight. Cramping & borborygmi possible. **Constipation**. Steatorrhea. Severe symptoms.
(c)	O	O	X	O	Delayed borborygmi and delayed hard to detect, mild, bloating that disappears overnight. Cramping possible. **Constipation.**
(d)	X	O	X	O	Delayed borborygmi and delayed hard to detect, mild, bloating that disappears overnight. Cramping possible. **Constipation.** Steatorrhea. Severe symptoms.
(e)	O	X	X	O	Immediate borborygmi and immediate hard to detect, mild, bloating that disappears overnight. Cramping possible. **Constipation.**
(f)	X	X	X	O	Immediate borborygmi and immediate hard to detect, mild, bloating that disappears overnight. Cramping possible. **Constipation.** Steatorrhea. Severe symptoms.

Legend: X = defective and O = functioning

Table 1. Summary of the six forms of IBS-C

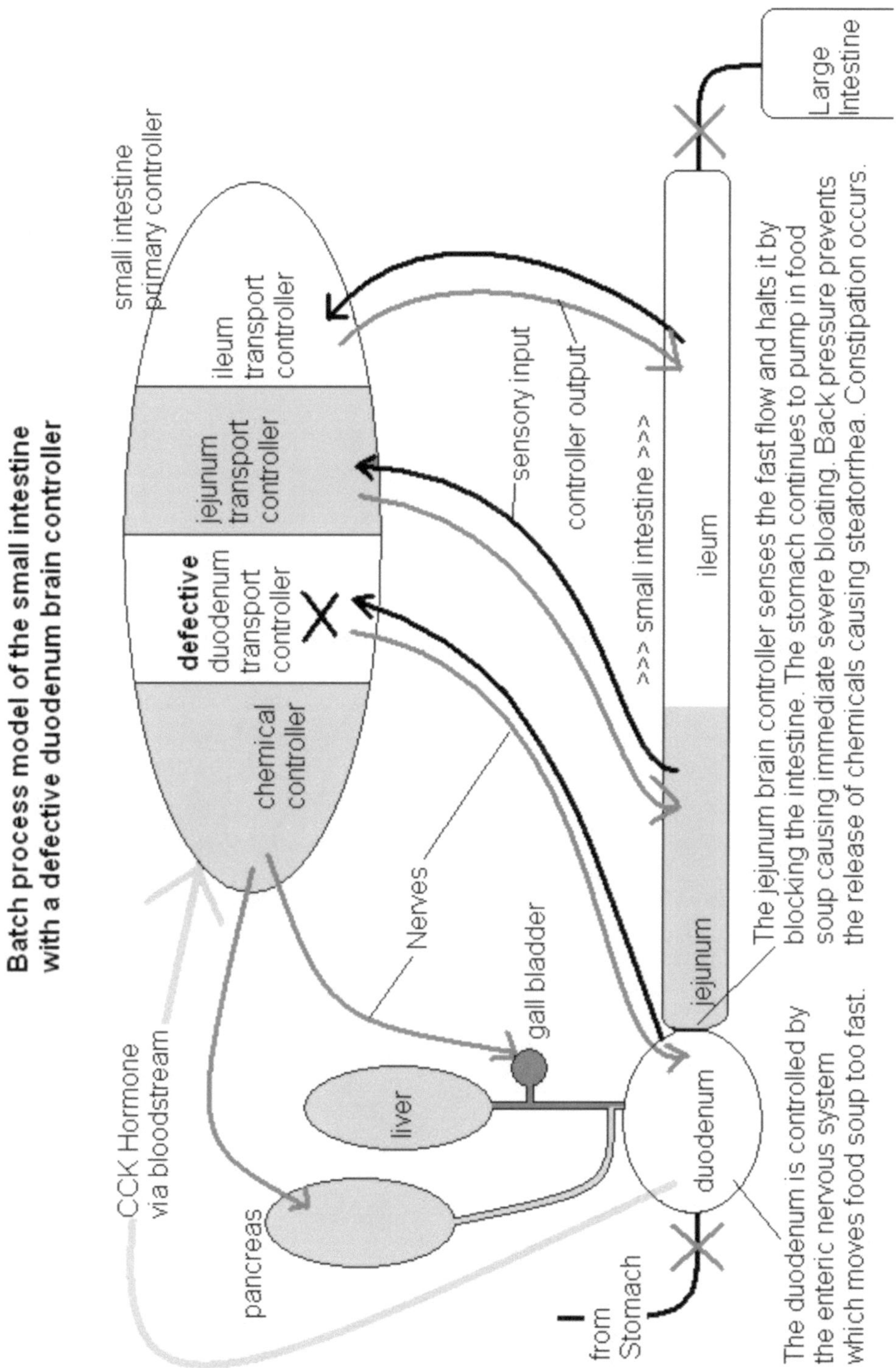

Diagram 1. Schematic showing how the model creates IBS-C form (a)

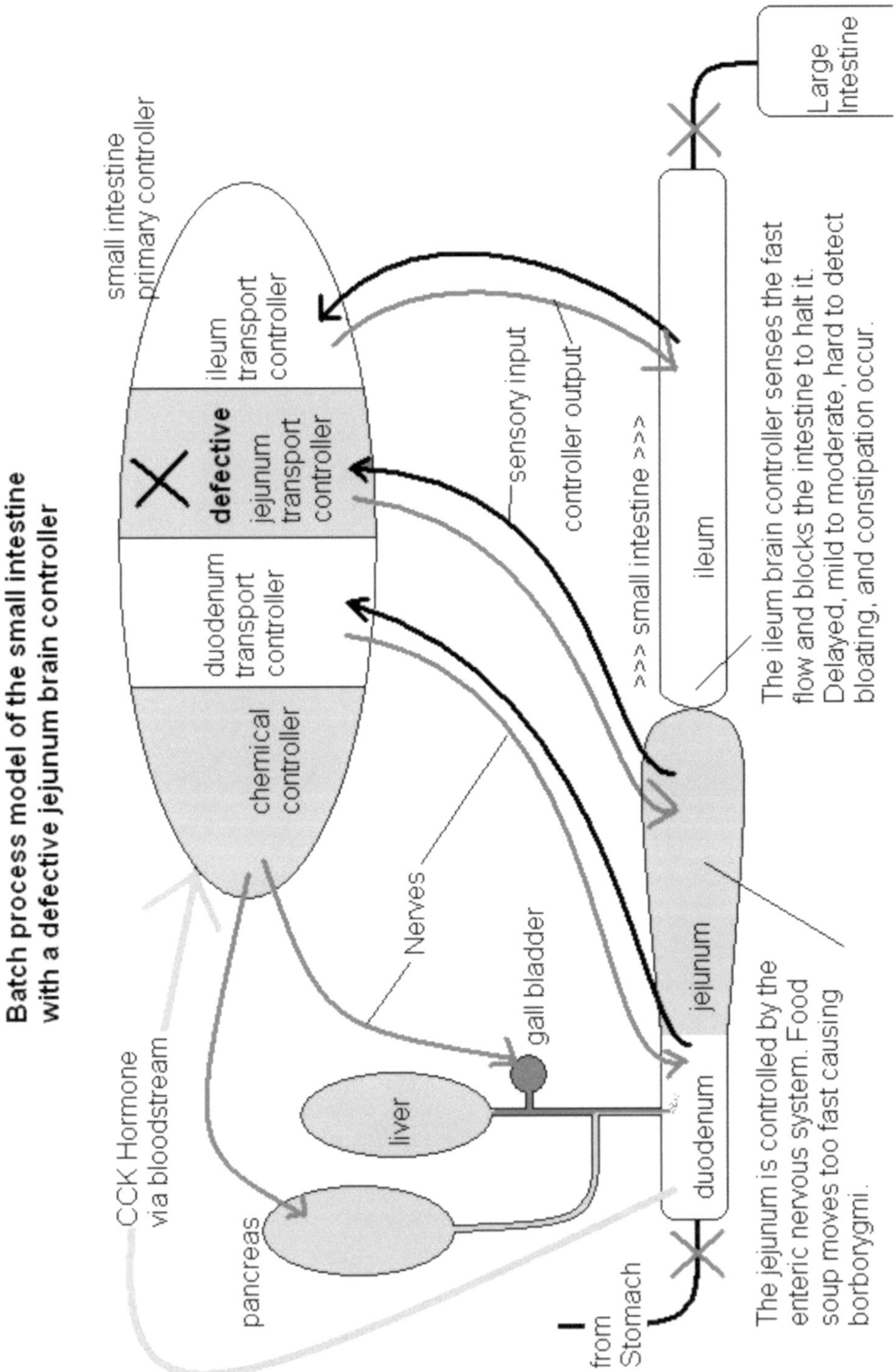

Diagram 2. Schematic showing how the model creates IBS-C form (c)

d. Form (c) as above together with IBS-B.
e. Both the duodenum and jejunum sub-controller outputs are deficient or missing. This causes a Barrier to form at the start of the ileum. When a breakfast containing cereal is eaten, borborygmi occurs followed by hard to detect, slight to moderate bloating. Onset of these symptoms is immediate.
f. Form (e) as above together with IBS-B.

3.6 The uncontrolled ileum - Diarrhoea

When the ileum is no longer correctly controlled by the primary transport controller, the secondary transport controller moves food soup at speed into the colon. The soup contains high levels of chemicals & possibly fats, and these cause automatic evacuation of the colon. The level of activity in the autonomic nervous system controls the valve at the end of the small intestine. When adrenal hormones are released on arising, the valve is easy to open, and the ileum immediately pushes its contents into the colon (the morning rush). When stress occurs during the day and releases adrenal hormones, the valve is again easier to open. Overnight the valve becomes more firmly closed. In severe cases of IBS-D & A, the ileum can push food soup through the valve at any time.

3.6.1 IBS-D caused by a neurotransmitter deficiency

There are six forms;

a. The ileum controller output is deficient or missing. When a breakfast containing cereal is eaten, borborygmi begin when food soup reaches the ileum several hours later. Diarrhoea occurs immediately after food soup reaches the end of the ileum or on arising (see Diagram 3).
b. Form (a) together with IBS-B.
c. The ileum and jejunum controller outputs are deficient or missing. When a breakfast containing cereal is eaten, borborygmi begin when food soup reaches the jejunum a few minutes later. Diarrhoea occurs immediately after food soup reaches the end of the ileum or on arising.
d. Form (c) together with IBS-B.
e. The ileum, jejunum and duodenum controller outputs are deficient or missing. When a breakfast containing cereal is eaten, borborygmi begin immediately. Diarrhoea occurs immediately after food soup reaches the end of the ileum or on arising.
f. Form (e) together with IBS-B.

3.6.2 IBS-A caused by a neurotransmitter deficiency

There are two forms;

a. The duodenum and ileum sub-controller outputs are deficient or missing. This causes IBS-C plus IBS-D. **Constipation** and diarrhoea alternate irregularly. The state of the autonomic nervous system controls the alternation.
b. Form (a) together with IBS-B.

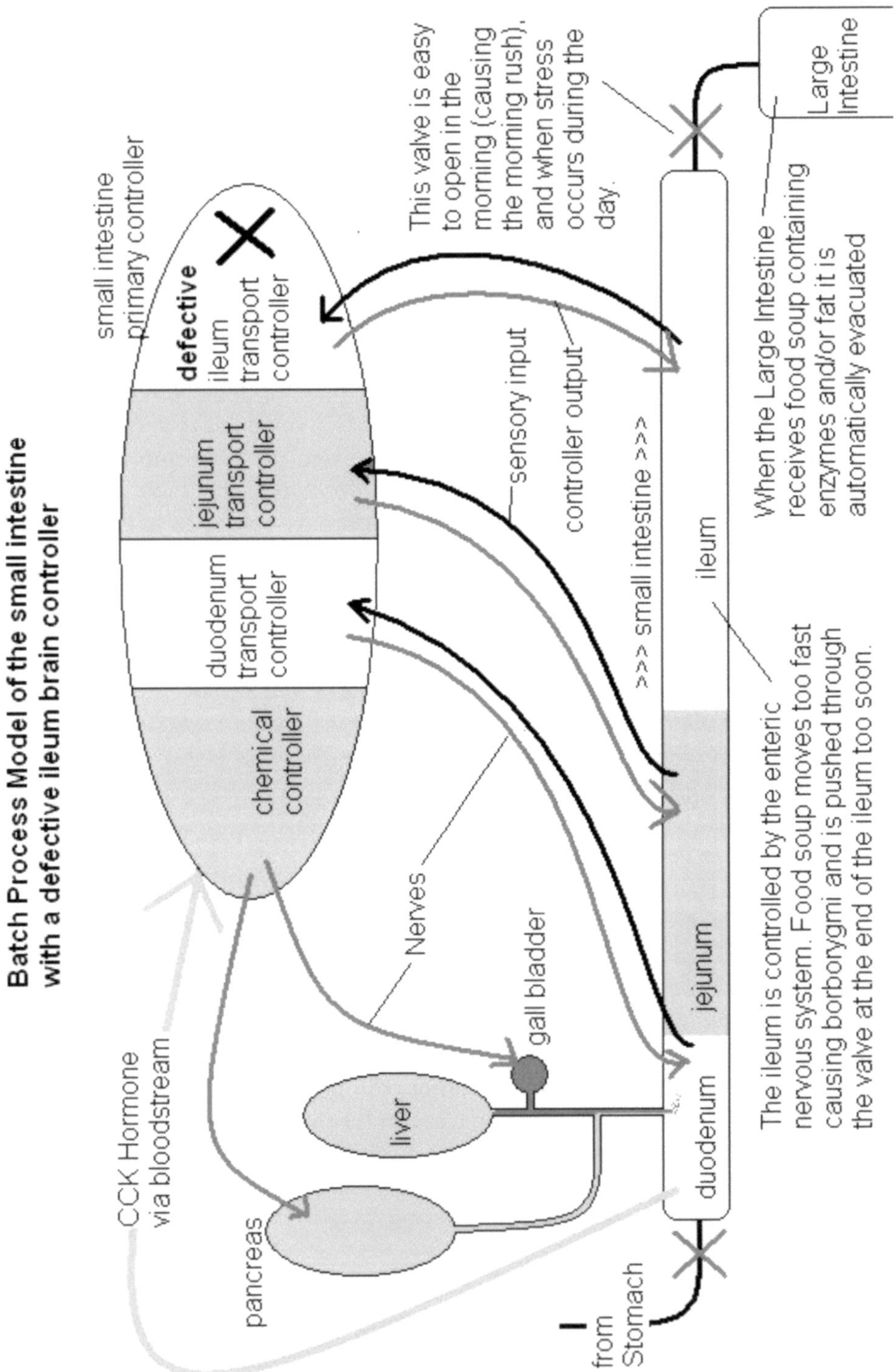

Diagram 3. Schematic showing how the model creates IBS-D form (a)

#	Primary controller				Symptoms
	Chemical	Duodenum	Jejunum	Ileum	
(a)	O	O	O	X	Borborygmi starting several hours after eating. Diarrhoea
(b)	X	O	O	X	Borborygmi starting several hours after eating. Diarrhoea. Steatorrhea. Severe symptoms.
(c)	O	O	X	X	Borborygmi starting a short time after eating. Diarrhoea
(d)	X	O	X	X	Borborygmi starting a short time after eating. Diarrhoea. Steatorrhea. Severe symptoms.
(e)	O	X	X	X	Borborygmi starting immediately after eating. Diarrhoea.
(f)	X	X	X	X	Borborygmi starting immediately after eating. Diarrhoea. Steatorrhea. Severe symptoms.

Legend: X = defective and O = functioning

Table 2. Summary of the six forms of IBS-D

#	Primary controller				Symptoms
	Chemical	Duodenum	Jejunum	Ileum	
(a)	O	X	O	X	**Constipation** & diarrhoea that alternate. Cramping, borborygmi, steatorrhea and severe bloating are possible.
(b)	X	X	O	X	**Constipation** & diarrhoea that alternate. Steatorrhea causes severe diarrhoea. Cramping, borborygmi and severe bloating are possible.

Legend: X = defective and O = functioning

Table 3. Summary of the two forms of IBS-A

3.7 Primary control fault summary

#	Primary controller				IBS Type(s)
	Chemical	Duodenum	Jejunum	Ileum	
1	X	O	O	O	B
2	O	X	O	O	C
3	X	X	O	O	C, B
4	O	O	X	O	C
5	X	O	X	O	C, B
6	O	X	X	O	C
7	X	X	X	O	C, B
8	O	O	O	X	D
9	X	O	O	X	D, B
10	O	O	X	X	D
11	X	O	X	X	D, B
12	O	X	X	X	D
13	X	X	X	X	D, B
14	O	X	O	X	A
15	X	X	O	X	A, B

Legend: X = defective and O = functioning

Table 4. Summary of the four types and fifteen forms of IBS produced when neurotransmitter deficiencies occur in the primary controller.

3.8 Other primary control faults

Any fault that disrupts sensory input from the small intestine to the brain or motor output from the brain to the small intestine will cause IBS symptoms. The section(s) of the intestine that are affected will not be the same as when a neurotransmitter is deficient. The first faulty section will cause an IBS Barrier to form at the start of the following brain controlled section. Subsequent defects will have little effect, except that diarrhoea symptoms will occur when a section that terminates the intestine is faulty. IBS-B cannot be produced by damage to the duodenum walls.

4. Variation in the expression of IBS symptoms

If you compare two subjects with the same type of IBS, the symptoms that they each suffer from can be different. The following factors explain how this variation occurs.

4.1 Food variables

When the enteric nervous system controls movement of food soup in the small intestine, the transport speed varies according to the types of food eaten. Some foods cause very fast speeds and others slower speeds.

More force is used to achieve very fast speeds, and the brain creates a stronger Barrier to stop the flow. A strong Barrier produces a complete transport halt for long periods, and dehydration occurs prematurely. This causes later processes of the small intestine to take longer. **Constipation**, bloating & cramping are increased in severity.

On arising, the valve at the end of the ileum is easy to open, and fast speeds in the ileum trigger the 'morning rush'. Very fast speeds move food into the colon immediately it reaches the end of the ileum.

Cramping occurs when the speed of food is too fast, and a Barrier is formed with its associated bloating. This is the enteric nervous system attempting to force food though the Barrier.

Cramping also occurs when the intestinal muscles are moving food at speed, in any part of the intestine. This cramping is accompanied by loud borborygmi.

When the colon receives food soup from the ileum that contains fat and/or high levels of digestive enzymes, it evacuates at speed, often with cramping.

4.1.1 Fibre

Some fibre types stimulate fast speeds in the small intestine when the secondary controller is active. Fast speeds cause slight to moderate IBS symptoms and very fast speeds cause severe IBS symptoms. Other types of fibre stimulate slower speeds. Data on the transport speed of different foods, when the enteric nervous system is in control of the small intestine, is in Table 5.

Food	*Speed*		*Food*	*Speed*
Wholemeal cereal flours	supersonic		Dahls (hulled split legumes)	slow
Whole cereals	very fast		Vegetables	slow
White cereal flours	fast		Fruits	slow
Polished cereals	fast		Animal foods	slow
Whole legumes	supersonic		Nuts and seeds	slow

Table 5. Speed of food types when transported by the enteric nervous system.

The outer coat of legumes and most cereals contain the fibre types that stimulate fast speeds in the small intestine. This fibre can be classed as insoluble, but not all types of insoluble fibre stimulate fast speeds.

4.1.2 Examination of fibre from cereals and legumes

1. *Whole wheat flour*...this food causes severe IBS symptoms. Insoluble fibre was extracted from whole wheat flour (machine ground), by boiling in 3% hydrochloric acid for several hours. The fibre consisted of 'two dimensional' flakes of bran with sharply defined edges, ranging in size from 2mm to 0.01mm (see Figures 1, 2 & 3).
2. *Whole white rice*...this food causes slight to moderate symptoms of IBS. Insoluble fibre was extracted from polished rice by cooking, then crushing and boiling in 3% hydrochloric acid for several hours. The fibre consisted of large 'two dimensional' flat sheets with sharply defined edges, ranging in size from 2mm to 5mm (see Figure 4).

3. *Corn grits…* this food causes no IBS symptoms. Insoluble fibre was extracted by boiling coarse corn meal (machine ground) in 3% hydrochloric acid for several hours. At 40x magnification the fibre consisted of three dimensional amorphous clumps and fragments (see Figure 5). The fibre appears to be tangled clumps of soft fibrils at 400x magnification (see Figure 6).
4. *Split yellow peas…* this food causes no IBS symptoms. Insoluble fibre was extracted from hulled & split yellow peas by soaking overnight, crushing, and then boiling in 3% hydrochloric acid for several hours. The insoluble material was obloid and spherical lumps, 0.1 to 0.3 mm in diameter (see Figures 7 & 8). Sharp edges were not visible.
5. *Haricot bean endosperm (internal portion)…* this food causes no IBS symptoms. Insoluble fibre was extracted by soaking whole beans overnight, removing the external coat, and boiling the crushed endosperm in 3% hydrochloric acid for several hours. The insoluble material was obloid and spherical lumps, 0.1 to 0.2 mm in diameter (see Figures 9 & 10). Sharp edges were not visible.
6. *Haricot bean external coat…* this food causes severe IBS symptoms. Insoluble fibre was extracted by soaking whole beans overnight, removing the external coat, crushing it and boiling in 3% hydrochloric acid for several hours. The fibre consisted of flat two dimensional fragments about 1 to 5 mm in size (see Figure 11). At 400x magnification the material is seen to be composed of densely packed crystalline rods, about 0.03mm long and 0.01mm in diameter (see Figure 12). The rods are orientated at 90 degrees to the surface of the endosperm.
7. *Moong bean endosperm…* this food causes no IBS symptoms. Insoluble fibre was extracted by soaking whole beans overnight, removing the external coat, and boiling the crushed endosperm in 3% hydrochloric acid for several hours. The fibre consisted of obloid to spherical lumps, 0.1 to 0.2 mm in diameter (see Figure 13). Sharp edges were not visible.
8. *Moong bean external coat…* this food causes moderate IBS symptoms. Insoluble fibre was extracted by soaking beans overnight, removing the skin, crushing and then boiling it in 3% hydrochloric acid for several hours. The fibre is fragments of light coloured coat with dark veins (see Figure 14). The dark veins contain crystalline rods orientated like the sleepers on a railway track (see Figure 15). Figure 16 shows 0.05mm by 0.01mm rods removed from the dark veins.

4.1.3 Insoluble fibre

Currently all insoluble fibre is treated the same. This research has identified three distinct types of insoluble fibre;

1. *Cereal bran…* sharp edged, two dimensional flakes present in most cereals. It causes severe IBS symptoms when present in quantity.
2. *Legume micro-crystalline fibre...* these tiny, hard, crystalline rods are found in the external coats of legumes. In high numbers they trigger severe IBS symptoms.
3. *Soft insoluble fibre…* Soft amorphous material from corn, legumes, fruits, vegetables, nuts, seeds & animal foods. It caused no IBS symptoms.

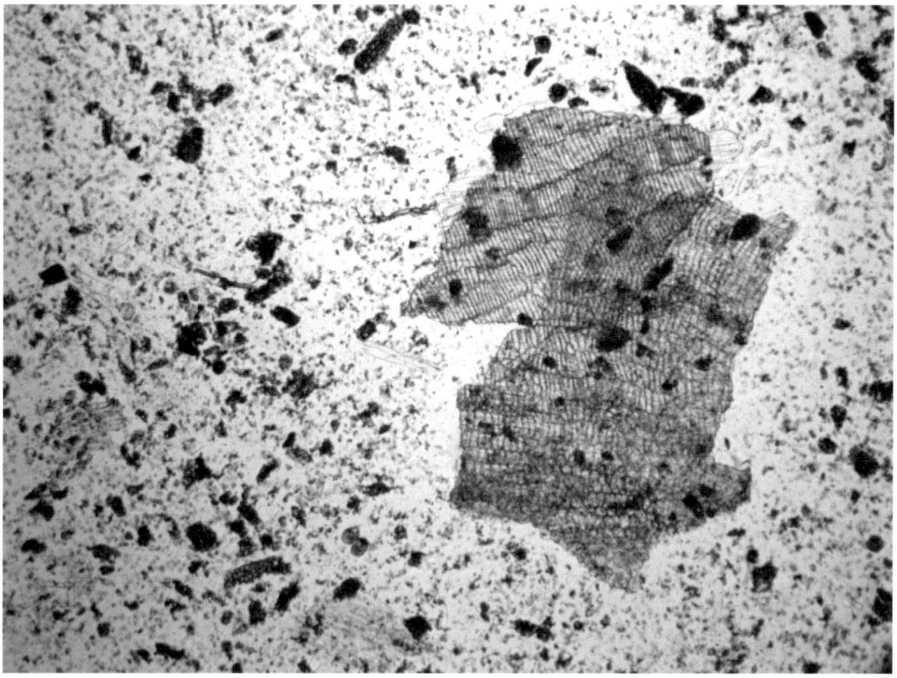

Fig. 1. Insoluble fibre from whole meal wheat flour x 40. Image 3mm wide.

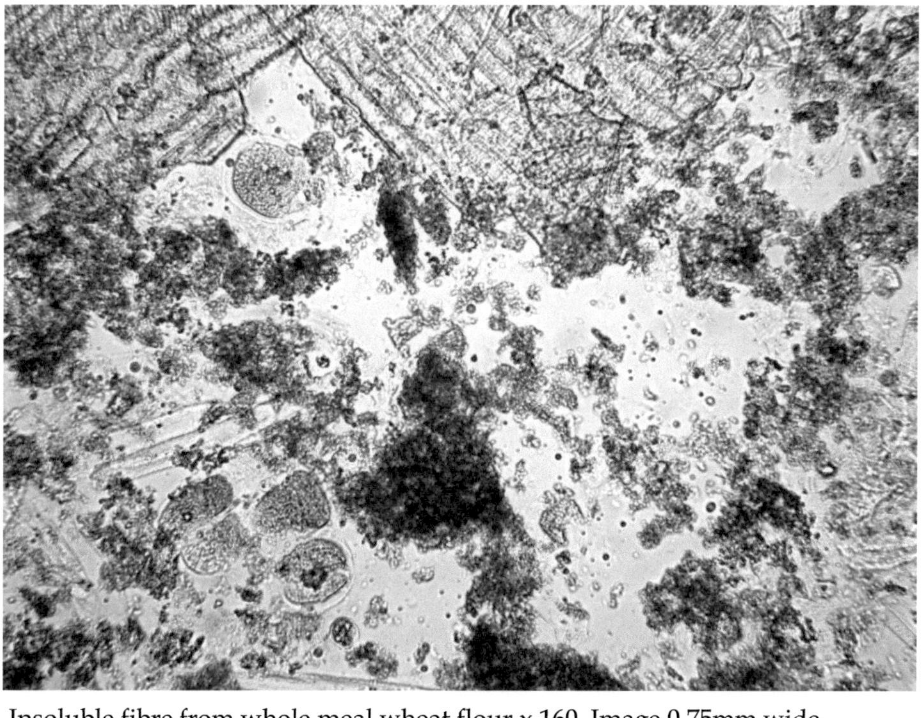

Fig. 2. Insoluble fibre from whole meal wheat flour x 160. Image 0.75mm wide

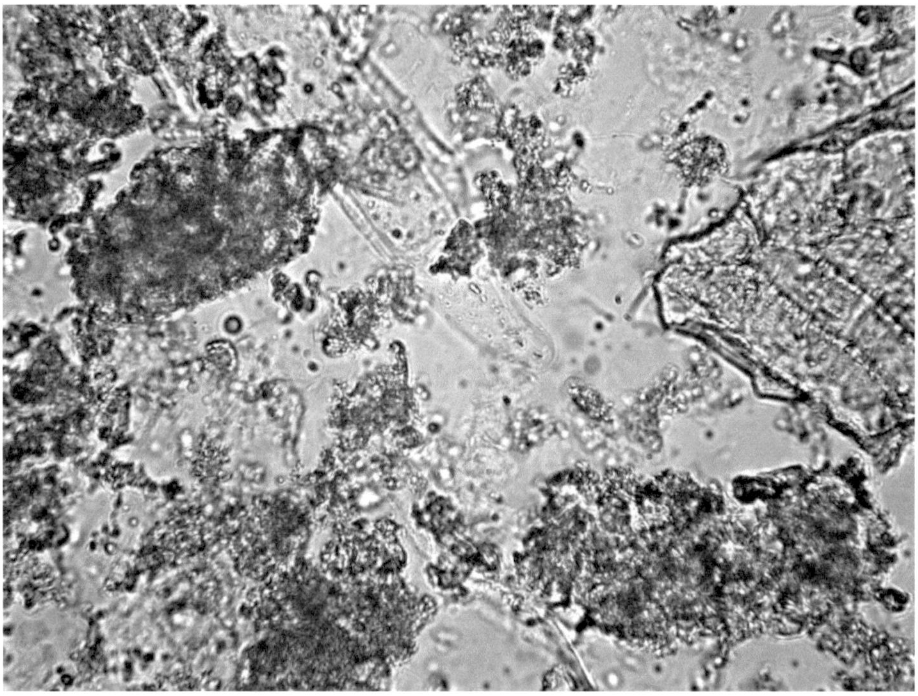

Fig. 3. Insoluble fibre from whole meal wheat flour x 400. Image 0.3mm wide

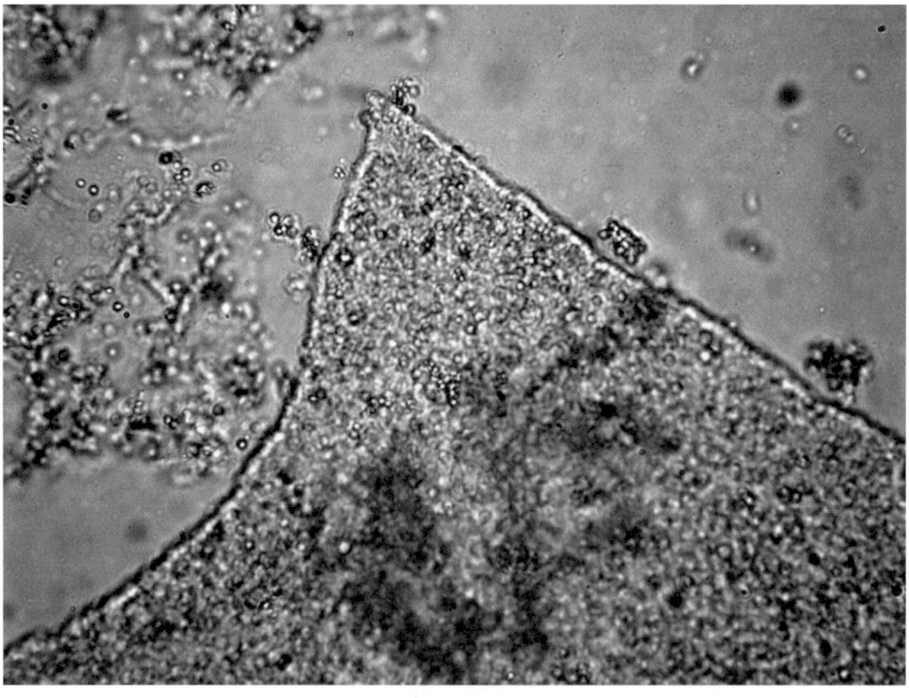

Fig. 4. Insoluble fibre from whole white rice x 400. Image 0.3mm wide

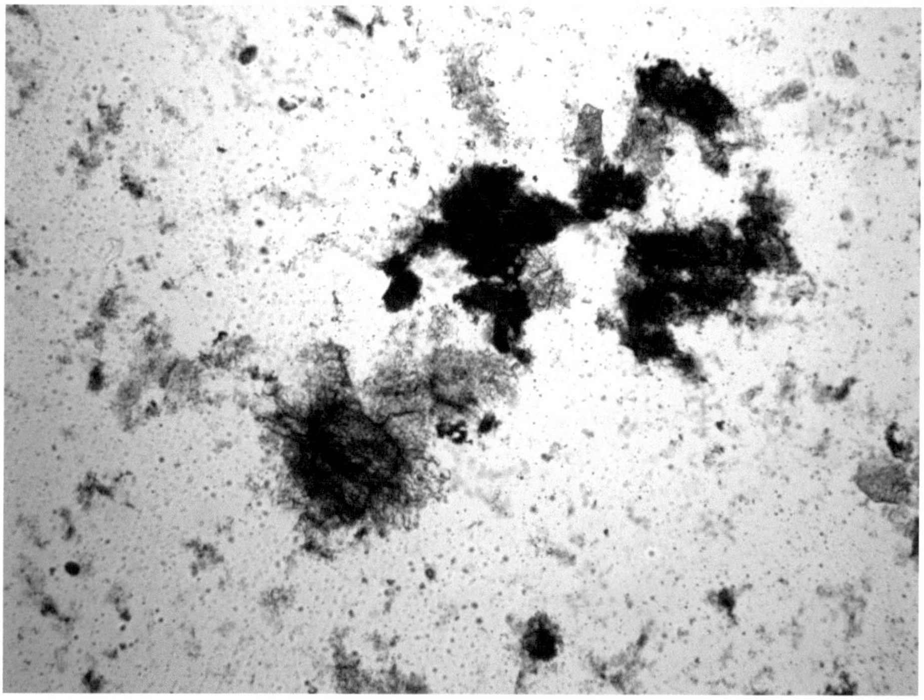

Fig. 5. Insoluble fibre extracted from corn grits x 40. Image 3mm wide.

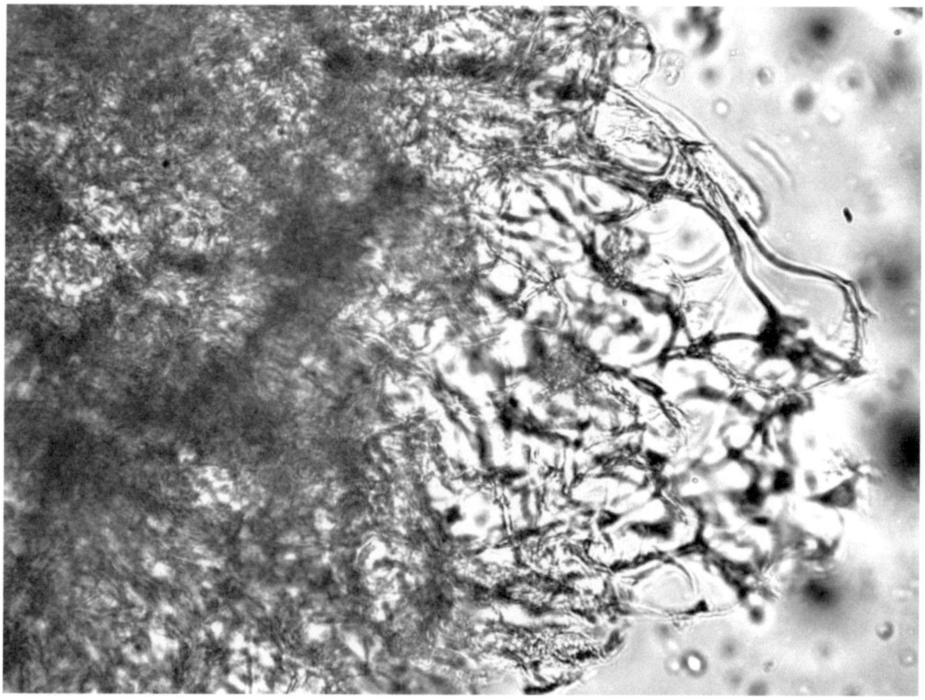

Fig. 6. Insoluble fibre extracted from corn grits x 400. Image 0.3mm wide.

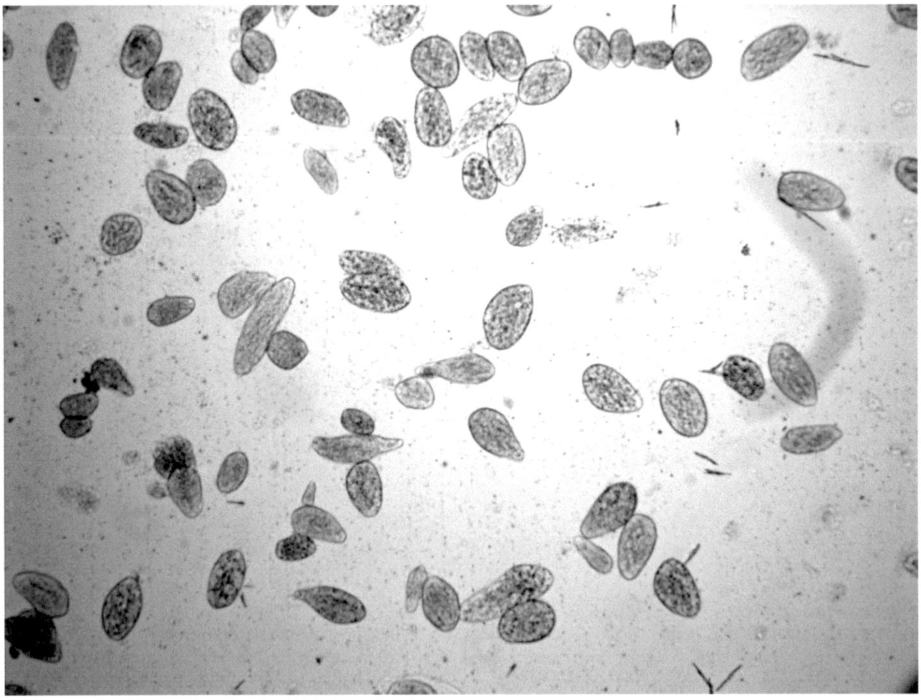

Fig. 7. Insoluble fibre from split yellow peas x 40. Image 3mm wide.

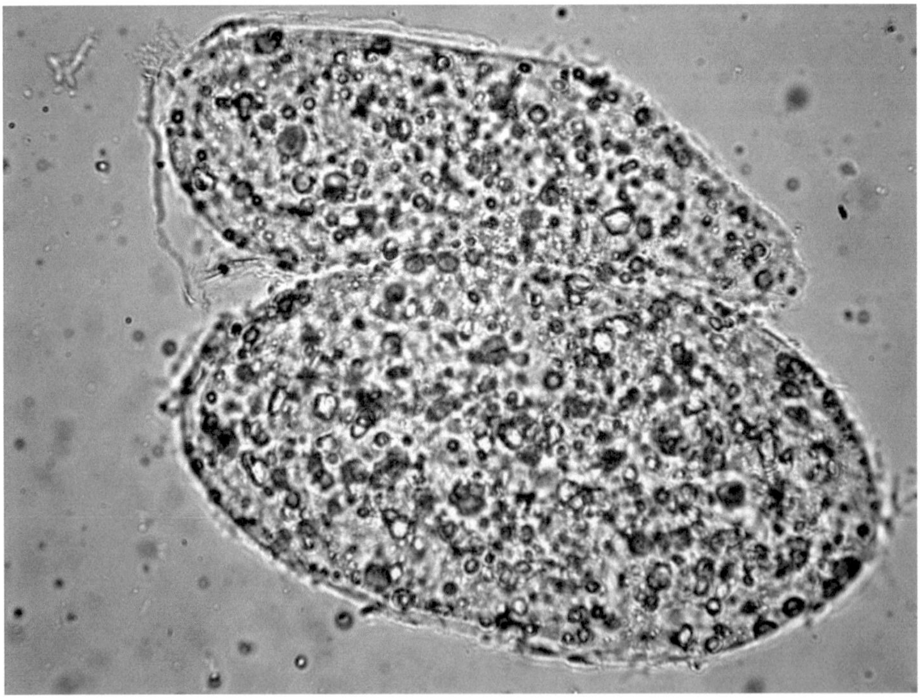

Fig. 8. Insoluble fibre from split yellow peas x 400. Image 0.3mm wide.

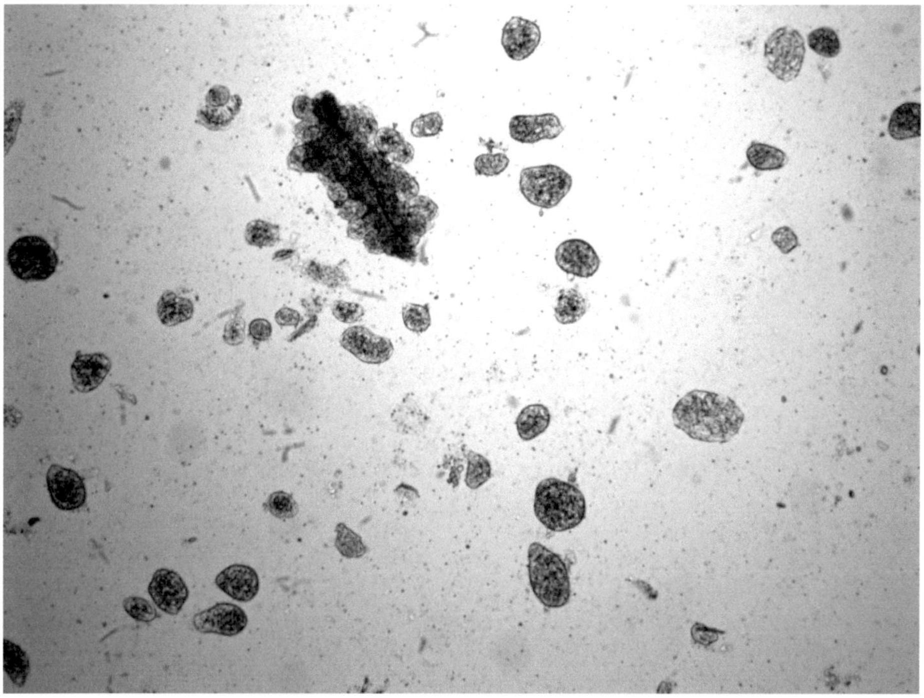

Fig. 9. Insoluble fibre from haricot bean endosperm x 40. Image 3mm wide.

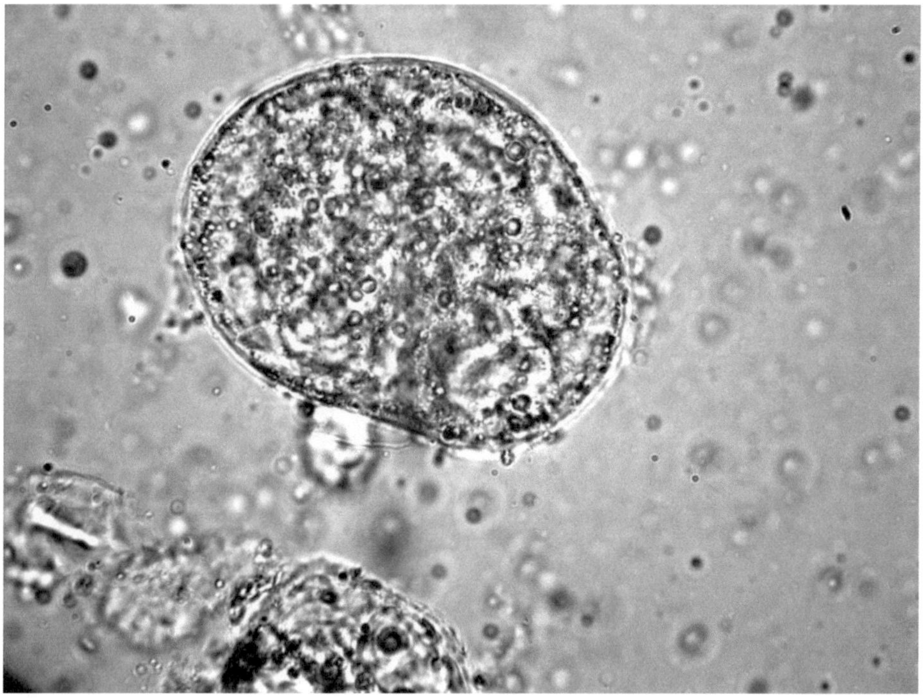

Fig. 10. Insoluble fibre from haricot bean endosperm x 400. Image 0.3mm wide.

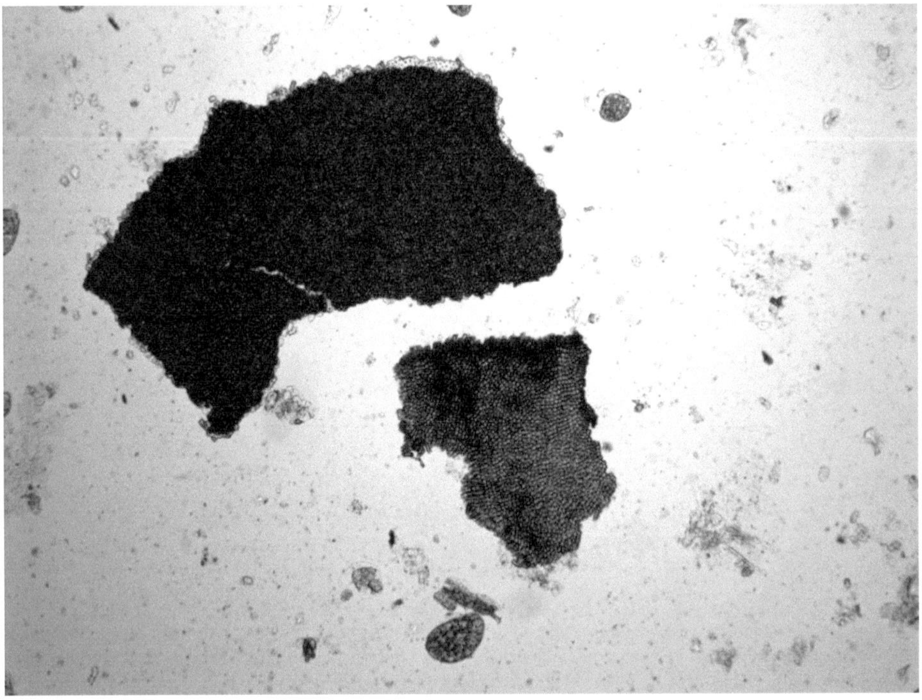

Fig. 11. Insoluble fibre from haricot bean external coat x 40. Image 3mm wide.

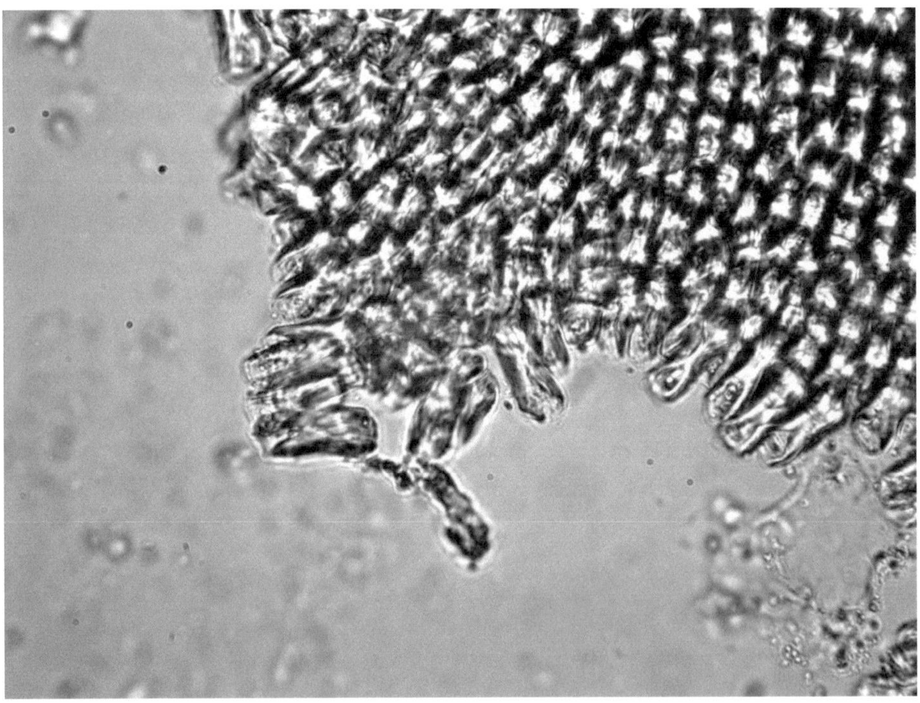

Fig. 12. Insoluble fibre from haricot bean external coat x 400. Image 0.3mm wide.

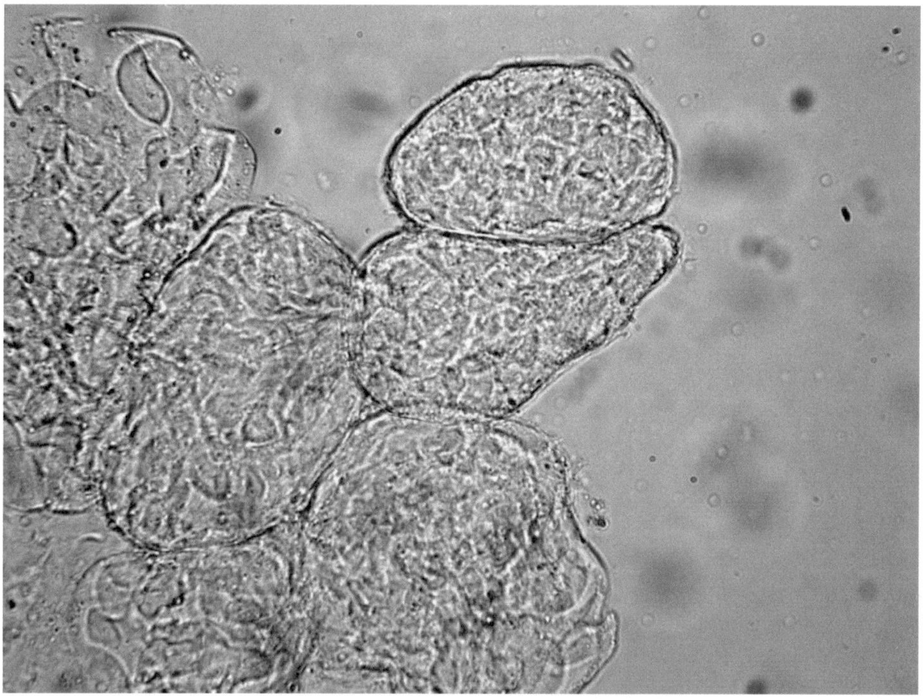

Fig. 13. Insoluble fibre from moong bean endosperm x 400. Image 0.3mm wide.

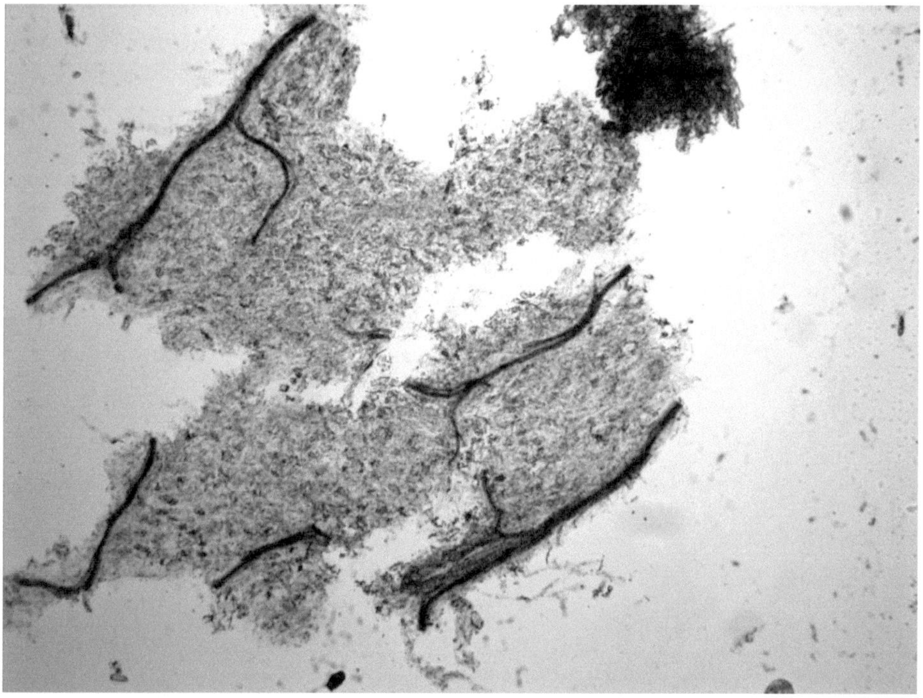

Fig. 14. Insoluble fibre from moong bean external coat x 40. Image 3mm wide.

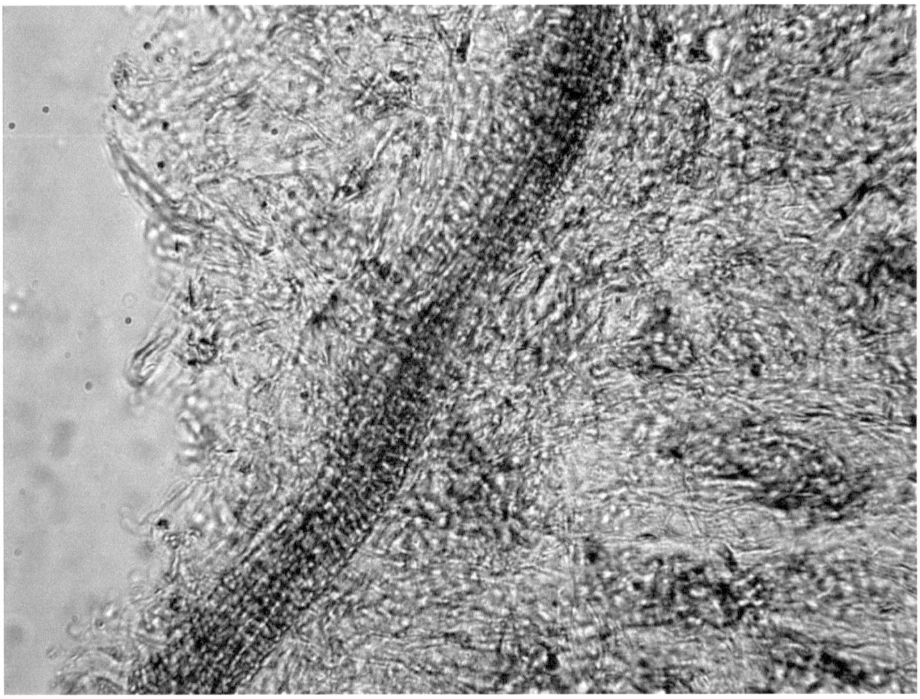

Fig. 15. Insoluble fibre from moong bean external coat x 400. Image 0.3mm wide.

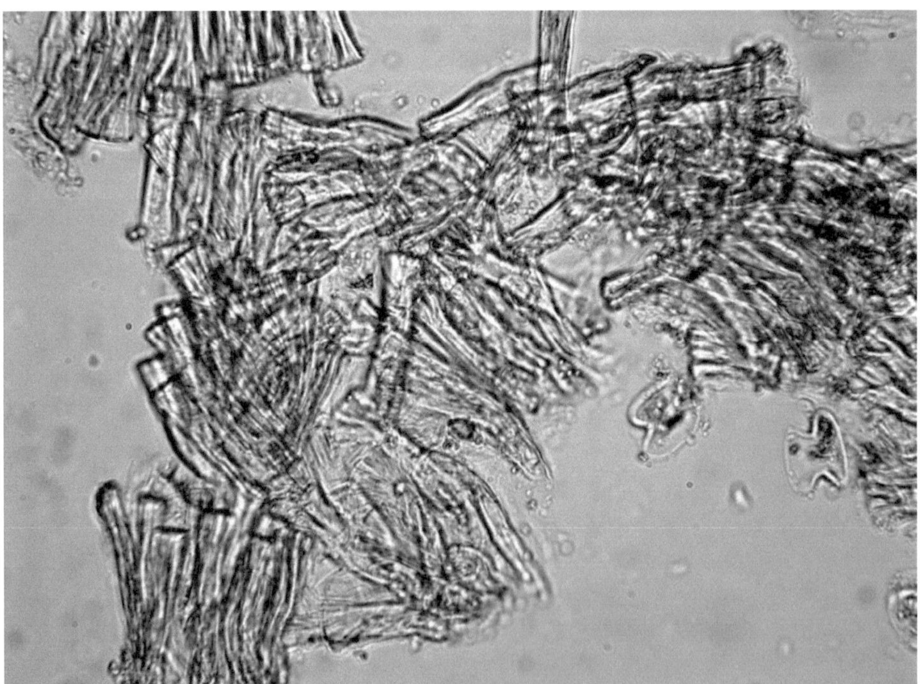

Fig. 16. Insoluble fibre from moong bean external coat x 400. Image 0.3mm wide.

4.1.4 Foods that slow the digestive system

Some foods reduce the speed of the digestive system. This allows more time for dehydration to occur. Their effects are not seen when cereals and whole legumes are eaten. The foods are...

- Cooked protein foods... chemicals called heterocyclic amines (HCAs) are formed when proteins are cooked. These can have an anaesthetic action in the digestive system.
- Dairy foods have refrigerant properties that slow the digestive system. They also contain opioid peptides that slow the digestive system.
- Gluten is a protein found in some cereals. It contains opioid peptides that can slow the digestive system. It also causes leaky bowel syndrome (Fasano & Shea-Donohue, 2005).
- Fruits that are astringent can slow the digestive system by drying it up.
- Spices can dehydrate the digestive system and slow it down.

4.1.5 Trace minerals and depression

When a high starch, low fat, cooked protein diet is eaten, trace minerals are supplied by the bacteria that digest residual starch & protein in the colon. These bacteria transform inorganic trace minerals into absorbable organic trace mineral complexes. However in IBS-A & IBS-D, colonic bacteria are regularly expelled and no longer supply trace minerals. Lack of these minerals causes depression.

4.2 Cholesterol

The human body manages circulating cholesterol with the ileum. Cholesterol is used to make bile salts which are then stored in the gall bladder. This removes cholesterol from circulation. Bile salts are used to emulsify fats in the first and second sections of the small intestine and later on they can be reabsorbed in the third section (ileum). The ileum brain controller manages this recycling process. When cholesterol level is low, most bile salts are recycled. When cholesterol level is high, more bile salts are allowed to escape via the stool.

- IBS-B... here the chemical addition brain controller's ability to release bile salts from the gall bladder is restricted, and the gall bladder becomes full. Excess cholesterol can no longer be reduced by making bile salts.
- IBS-A & IBS-D... here the ileum brain controller's ability to manage the recycling of bile salts is compromised. Large amounts can be lost. Circulating cholesterol is diverted to bile salt manufacture, and a cholesterol deficit can occur.

4.2.1 Symptoms of cholesterol deficit & excess

When the ability to eliminate cholesterol via the digestive process is compromised, a high level of cholesterol causes the brain to display characteristic symptoms. When excessive amounts of bile salts are lost because of a defective ileum, a low cholesterol level causes similar symptoms. They are...

1. Visual hallucinations... these are kaleidoscopic moving patterns of colour that start near the centre of the visual field and radiate outwards. They are followed by...
2. Headaches and impaired brain function.

4.3 Variable level of the autonomic nervous system

The level of the autonomic nervous system is high on arising and when environmental stress occurs. Overnight it usually declines. This variation coincides with levels of adrenal hormones in the body. Now the small intestine is controlled by five divisions of the autonomic nervous system. Variation in the activity level of this system thus affects control of the small intestine. IBS symptoms are worst early in the morning. The characteristic IBS-A & D symptom of the 'morning rush' occurs when the enteric nervous system relaxes the valve terminating the ileum, moves the contents of the ileum prematurely into the colon, and evacuates the colon in response to the presence of raw enzymes and/or fat. The characteristic IBS-C & A symptom of bloating is worst on eating breakfast. The control speed set by the enteric nervous system is higher, and the strength of the Barrier is stronger.

4.4 Climate, age & constitution

- Living at arctic latitudes worsens symptoms, at tropical latitudes they improve.
- IBS is seldom severe in young people. IBS is often severe in old age.
- Some constitutions suffer more from IBS. Those that suffer most are thin and underweight. Substantial constitutions cope better.

4.5 Progression of the illness

A neurotransmitter deficiency (or deficiencies) in the small intestine brain controller, can develop over decades. IBS symptoms are mild and irregular at first, gradually become more frequent, then continuous.

4.6 Other causes of IBS

- Severing of nerves during surgery to the abdomen will cause symptoms immediately.
- Damage to the intestine from a toxic insult will cause symptoms immediately.
- Pressure on nerves in the neck area from misaligned vertebrae, will cause intermittent symptoms.
- Damage to intestinal nerves from pregnancy or childbirth, will result in immediate symptoms.
- Failure of nervous system development as an infant will cause symptoms to appear as soon as solid foods are fed.

5. Evidence for the model

5.1 No visible damage

Medical examination of most IBS patients shows no damage that can account for the symptoms. The automated controls of the digestive system are where the problems are likely to be.

5.2 Cereal and legume fibre

When consumption of cereals and whole legumes is stopped, IBS symptoms are dramatically improved. These foods stimulate too fast speeds when the enteric nervous system regulates transport in the small intestine.

5.3 Difficulty digesting fats

The model identifies three possible causes of fat in the stool (steatorrhea)...

1. When severe bloating is a symptom, backpressure in the duodenum prevents the release of sufficient chemicals.
2. When a defective ileum causes continual diarrhoea, large amounts of chemicals can be lost. The gall bladder and pancreas no longer contain enough chemicals.
3. IBS-B explains the other cases of impaired fat digestion. Here the brain can no longer release enough chemicals.

5.4 Irritation around the anus

Diarrhoea is often accompanied by irritation of the skin around the anus. When the ileum no longer efficiently recycles chemicals, bowel movements will contain raw protease enzymes. These attack the area around the anus.

5.5 Intestinal bloating

IBS bloating starts on arising when adrenal hormones are released and breakfast is eaten. Stress during the day further increases it. Overnight it can disappear. The autonomic nervous system is at a high level in the morning, high in response to stress and low overnight. It is likely to be causing the bloating.

The symptom of bloating displays two degrees. It is either severe, or slight to moderate and hard to detect. The duodenum is short (25 cm). When the Barrier is at the start of the jejunum and the stomach continues to pump in food soup, bloating is severe (see Diagram 1). The jejunum is 2-3m long. When the Barrier is at the start of the ileum, it causes only slight to moderate bloating (see Diagram 2) that is hard to detect.

5.6 Intestinal cramping

1. Cramping associated with bloating is the secondary transport controller trying to move food soup through a Barrier created by a primary transport controller. It pushes in one direction only (forward). The strength of the pushing depends on the type of food eaten, and the state of the autonomic nervous system.
2. Cramping associated with loud borborygmi is the secondary transport controller moving food soup too fast in the small intestine.
3. Cramping followed immediately by diarrhoea, occurs when the secondary transport controller causes the ileum to move food soup into the colon too soon. The soup contains enzymes and/or fat, and the colon is evacuated immediately at speed.

6. Suggestions for testing the model

6.1 Three kinds of IBS-C

Clinicians may be able to find the three kinds of neurotransmitter deficient IBS-C predicted by the hypothesis.

1. The duodenum brain controller is deficient. When a breakfast containing cereal is eaten, the symptoms are immediate severe bloating and possibly cramping. **Constipation** and steatorrhea occur.
2. The jejunum brain controller is deficient. When a breakfast containing cereal is eaten, symptoms are borborygmi, and hard to detect, slight to moderate bloating, both delayed by a few minutes. **Constipation** occurs. Cramping and steatorrhea are possible.
3. Both the duodenum and jejunum brain controllers are deficient. When a breakfast containing cereal is eaten, symptoms are immediate borborygmi, and immediate slight to moderate bloating that is hard to detect. **Constipation** occurs. Cramping and steatorrhea are possible.

6.2 Three kinds of IBS-D

The symptom of borborygmi may allow the clinician to find the three kinds of neurotransmitter deficient IBS-D predicted by the theory. If IBS-B occurs, this may cause borborygmi that will obscure the diagnosis.

1. The ileum brain controller is malfunctioning. Borborygmi will start several hours after a breakfast containing cereal is eaten. Diarrhoea occurs immediately food reaches the end of the ileum, or on arising the next morning. Cramping and steatorrhea are possible.
2. Both the ileum and jejunum brain controllers are malfunctioning. Borborygmi will begin a few minutes after starting to eat a breakfast containing cereal. Diarrhoea occurs immediately food reaches the end of the ileum, or on arising the next morning. Cramping and steatorrhea are possible.
3. The ileum, jejunum, and duodenum brain controllers are malfunctioning. Borborygmi will begin immediately after starting to eat a breakfast containing cereal. Diarrhoea occurs immediately food reaches the end of the ileum, or on arising the next morning. Cramping and steatorrhea are possible.

7. Coping with IBS symptoms

7.1 Key symptoms for diagnosis

The often confusing collection of symptoms that IBS presents, can be made sense of by using the key diagnostic criteria presented in Table 6.

IBS Type	*Identifying diagnostic symptoms*
IBS-A	Diarrhoea AND bloating
IBS-B	Steatorrhea often accompanied by severe symptoms of IBS-A, C, or D.
IBS-C	**Constipation** but NO diarrhoea
IBS-D	Diarrhoea but NO bloating.

Table 6. Diagnostic criteria for IBS

Diagnosis of IBS-B may cause problems, as steatorrhea can also be caused by continual diarrhoea that empties the gall bladder & pancreas, and by backpressure in the duodenum. If diarrhoea & severe bloating are absent, and steatorrhea is present, then IBS-B is indicated. The presence of severe symptoms is also indicative of IBS-B. However dietary trials are likely to be needed to find out if IBS-B is definitely present.

7.2 Healing the symptoms

IBS symptoms are dramatically reduced by removing cereals and whole legumes from the diet (Dobson, 2011; Sinclair 2003). Most remaining symptoms can be removed with Relaxation Therapies. When stress releases adrenal hormones, the autonomic nervous system moves to a higher level, and IBS symptoms become worse. A cascade occurs…

Stress → IBS → more Stress → severe IBS etc…

Relaxation Therapies (Blanchard 1993, 2001; Dobson 2011), keep the level of adrenal hormones lower and the autonomic nervous system operates at a lower level. The enteric nervous system then moves food soup slower, the Barrier diminishes, and the valve into the colon is harder to open.

8. Future research

The author is currently developing a range of diets to treat IBS. The hypothesis presented here, together with the diets and relaxation therapies, will eventually be published in a book written so that all can understand.

More research…

- Location of the small intestine controllers in the brain.
- Identification of the four neurotransmitters in the small intestine brain controller.
- Identification of the receptor for the hormone Cholecystokinin in the small intestine chemical controller.

9. Acknowledgement

Thanks to Wai, Carol, Robert, Brenda, Bill, Pat, Celine, Janette, Andrea, Alwyn, Mark, Amanda, Paul, Lois, Alice, Miao, Carlos, Don Juan, Sw. Satyananda, & Elsevier, for their assistance. The facilities of the University of Auckland have also been very helpful.

10. References

Blanchard E.B. et al., (1993), Relaxation training as a treatment for irritable bowel syndrome, *Biofeedback Self-Regulation,* Vol. 18, No. 3, pp. 125, ISSN: 0363-3586.

Blanchard E.B., (2001), *Irritable bowel syndrome: psychosocial assessment and treatment,* American Psychological Association, ISBN: 1557987300.

Dobson B.C., (2008), The small intestine and irritable bowel syndrome (IBS): A batch process model, *Medical Hypotheses* Vol. 71, No. 5, pp. 781, ISSN: 0306-9877.

Dobson B.C., (2011), *IBS Explained*, Brian C. Dobson, Retrieved from www.ibsexplained.com

Drossman D.A. ed., (2007), *The functional gastrointestinal disorders ROME III. 3rd ed.*, pp. 490, www.degnon.org ISBN: 0-9656837-5-3.

Fasano A. & Shea-Donohue T., (2005), The role of intestinal barrier function in the pathogenesis of gastrointestinal autoimmune diseases, *Nature Clinical Practice Gastroenterology & Hepatology*, Vol. 2, No. 9, pp 416, ISSN: 1759-5045

Rehfeld J.F., (2004), Cholecystokinin, *Bailliere's Clinical Endocrinology and Metabolism*, Vol. 18, No. 4, pp. 569, ISSN: 0950-351X

Schwetz I., Lin Chang, (2004), *Encyclopedia Gastroenterology,* pp. 467, Elsevier, ISBN: 978-0-12-386860-2

Sinclair C, (2003) *The IBS low starch diet*, Ninox Publishing, ISBN: 0-9582529-0-4, www.lowstarchdiet.net

6

Opioid Induced Constipation

Caterina Aurilio, Maria Caterina Pace, Vincenzo Pota and Pasquale Sansone
Department of Anesthesiological, Surgical and Emergency Science, Second University of Naples, Naples, Italy

1. Introduction

The prevalence of chronic pain in the adult population ranges from2 to 40 (1–3). The chronic use of opioids for the treatment of non-cancer pain is commonly encountered in clinical practice.

The American Society of the Interventional Pain Physicians has issued guidelines for appropriate use of opioids (4).

With the increased use of opioids, there are more patients presenting with opioid induced constipation (OIC) or opioid bowel dysfunction (OBD) (5,6).

The definitions of constipation include a reference to infrequent, difficult or incomplete bowel evacuation that may lead to pain and discomfort; with stools that can range from small, hard 'rocks', to a large bulky mass. Constipation may be debilitating among those who require chronic analgesia (7); OIC or OBD affected an average of 41 % patients taking an oral opioid for up to 8 weeks in a meta-analysis of 11 placebo-controlled, randomized studies in non-malignant pain (14). In a survey of patients taking opioid therapy for pain of non-cancer origin, who required laxative therapy, only 46 % of opioid-treated patients reported achieving the desired treatment results > 50 % of the time, in contrast to the reported satisfaction in 84 % of control subjects (8).

The prevalence of constipation was 46.9 % and chronic abdominal pain 58.2 % among 100 ambulatory patients with moderate-to-severe chronic non-cancer pain.

In the United States and European survey of 322 patients taking daily oral opioids and laxatives, 45 % of patients reported < 3 bowel movements per week, 81 % reported constipation, and 58 % straining, symptoms were most oft en reported as severe, had at least a moderate negative impact on overall quality of life and activities of daily living. The objectives of this narrative review are to summarize essential aspects of the epidemiology of opiate-induced constipation (OIC), summarize the effects of opiates on gastrointestinal functions that lead to constipation, evaluate pharmacological approaches to treat or prevent OIC.

2. Pathophysiology of opioid induced constipation

The opioid receptors identified as having effects on human gastrointestinal function are δ -, κ -, and μ -receptors. They all belong to the family of G-protein-coupled receptors, and inhibit adenylate cyclase. The m-receptors are the principal mediators of the analgesic action of endogenous and exogenous opioids as well as of the major side-effects, ie, sedation, bowel dysfunction, respiratory depression, and dependence. At the membrane level, they reduce neuronal excitability and neurotransmitter (acetylcholine) release (9) with an overall inhibitory effect on the neuron.

Opioid receptors are widely distributed in the central and peripheral nervous system, the intestinal musculature, and other tissues. In the gastrointestinal tract, μ-receptors are widely distributed in the submucosa (10), as well as in the ileal mucosa. They influence ion transport changes (11). While μ - and κ -opiate receptors are more representative in stomach and proximal colon (12).

The cause of constipation in opiate users is multi-factorial (13). Opioids interfere with normal gastrointestinal motility by delaying transit, stimulating non-propulsive motility, segmentation and tone, and stimulation of sphincters such as the pylorus and ileocecal sphincter (13) through their effects on enteric neurons (14). They can also stimulate the absorption of fluids, mainly by delayed transit, and by stimulating mucosal sensory receptors that activate a reflex arc that facilitates further fluid absorption (15,16). These multiple effects lead to OIC.

3. Pharmacological approach to OIC

3.1 μ-opioid receptor agonists

Tapentadol

Tapentadol HCI is a μ -opioid agonist that also inhibits norepinephrine reuptake (17). The analgesic effect is so a combination of two different mechanism. In different trials norepinephrine reuptake inhibition (e.g., with venlafaxine (18) and the α 2-adrenergic agonist clonidine (19, 20) are associated with reduced colonic or rectal sensation in response to distension. Moreover it seems that, because of the combined analgesic action of tapentadol , the pain control can be achieved with a relatively lower level of μ-opioid agonism, which therefore reduces the gastrointestinal adverse effects such as constipation. As an analgesic tapentadol has a more favorable gastrointestinal side-effect profile than the classic μ-opioid receptor agonist oxycodone (21).

However, there were substantially lower incidences of gastrointestinal-related adverse effects with tapentadol extended release than with oxycodone controlled release (22). Similarly, tapentadol extended release, 100– 250 mg b.i.d., effectively relieved moderate-to-severe chronic low back pain over 15 weeks with a better gastrointestinal tolerability than oxycodone HCl controlled release, 20 - 50 mg b.i.d. (23). Studies of the pharmacodynamic effects of tapentadol on gastric emptying and colonic transit would be of significant interest.

3.2 μ-opioid receptor antagonists

The main problem in using opioid antagonist for reversing the gastrointestinal adverse effects of opioid that the dose efficaciousness in reversing OIC may inhibit the analgesic effect of opioids, causing either opiate withdrawal symptoms or reversal of desirable analgesia.

Naloxone

Naloxone is a competitive antagonist at opioid receptors with much greater affinity for μ - than for κ - or δ -receptors. Naloxone blocks opioid intestinal receptors and has low systemic bioavailability (2%) due to a marked hepatic first-pass effect. In patients with chronic pain, oral naloxone improved symptoms of laxation (24), but because of its very narrow therapeutic index, doses that reverse gut symptoms can often cause reversal of analgesia (25). However, there has been a resurgence of interest in naloxone in a prolonged-release preparation, which shows evidence of analgesic efficacy and safety when used in combination with oxycodone (prolonged release) for moderate-to-severe chronic pain (26) and improved bowel function when compared with oral oxycodone (prolonged release) alone (27). This effiacy continues for up to 52 weeks in patients with non-cancer chronic pain (28).

Naltrexone extended release

There one open-label study that evaluated the safety of a combination of extended-release pellets of morphine sulfate with a sequestered naltrexone core (administered once or twice daily) in patients with chronic, moderate to-severe pain. The pain-relieving objectives of treatment were achieved using dosages of the combination that could be adjusted in accordance with the investigator' s best medical judgment. The median average daily dose of morphine over the course of study in the safety population was 58.6 mg. 465 patients received one or more doses, 160 completed the 12-month study: 30% of the discontinuations occurred in the first month, most often because of adverse events (23.7 %), nausea (5.4 %), constipation in (3.4 %), and vomiting in (2.6 %). Most of the 465 patients (81.3 %) experienced one or more adverse events, most commonly constipation (31.8%) or nausea (25.2%). Opiate withdrawal symptoms were mild and affected < 5% of patients during each week of the study (29). Form these data the authors concluded that combination does not resolve OBD.

3.3 Association of opioid agonist and antagonist

Oxycodone/Naloxone

A new oral formulation (oxycodone/naloxone, OXN) that combines prolonged-release oxycodone (PRO) and prolonged-release naloxone (PRN) was devel- oped. The ratio of 2:1 PRO to PRN was chosen for the new tablets, which have different strengths: 5/2.5 mg, 10/5 mg, 20/10 mg and 40/20 mg [30,31]. The aim of this formulation is to counteract opioid-induced con- stipation (OIC) development [32] through naloxone local antagonist effect on the opioid receptors in the gut wall [33] while maintain analgesia [35] due to the high systemic oxycodone availability after oral ad- ministration (60–87%)

Meissner et al. [30] reported a randomized, double- blind study that assessed analgesic efficacy and, impact on the OIC of OXN and identified the optimal dose ratio of oxycodone and naloxone. Two hundred and two patients with chronic pain (most non-malignant, 2.5% cancer-related pain) and stable oxycodone dose (40, 60 or 80 mg per day) were randomized into groups that received 10, 20, and 40 mg per day naloxone or placebo. After 4 weeks of the maintenance phase, patients received oxycodone for two weeks. Pain intensity was evaluated by the NRS, and bowel function was assessed by the bowel function index (BFI). No loss of analgesia with naloxone was observed. Na- loxone at doses of 20 and 40 mg improved bowel function in comparison to placebo ($p < 0.05$). The combination was well tolerated with no unexpected adverse effects. A trend towards an increase in diarrhea with the higher naloxone doses was observed. The 2:1 oxyco- done/naloxone ratio was identified as the most suitable.

3.4 Peripherally restricted μ- opiate receptor antagonists

Methylnaltrexone

Methylnaltrexone is a quaternary ammonium derivative of naltrexone, an opioid antagonist similar to naloxone, but it is less lipid soluble, so, less likely to cross the blood–brain barrier (36). Methylnaltrexone blocks acute morphine-induced delay in orocecal transit time without affecting analgesia or causing central opiate withdrawal symptoms.

Intravenous methylnaltrexone infusion reversed methadone induced constipation, increasing stool frequency and decreasing orocecal transit times (37,38). Orally administered methylnaltrexone showed the same results (39) with plasma drug levels were very low, suggesting a local site of action in the gut.

Several studies evaluated the effect of methylnaltrexone on apin and OIC. Methylnaltrexone, 0.45 mg / kg intravenously (i.v.), reversed the effects of 0.05 and 0.1 mg/kg morphine on orocecal transit in healthy volunteers (40)

Methylnaltrexone (at a dose of 0.15 mg / kg subcutaneously (s.c.), every other day for 2 weeks) was tested for OIC in advanced illness in 133 patients who had received opioids for 2 or more weeks and had received stable doses of opioids and laxatives for 3 or more days without relief of OIC (41). Methylnaltrexone s.c. has been approved by the US Food and Drug Administration, Health Canada and the European Medicines Agency (42). The approved indication is OIC in patients with advanced illness receiving palliative care after failing laxative therapy, and the usual dosing schedule is 1 dose every other day, as needed, but no more frequently than 1 dose in a 24-h period. The recommended dose of methylnaltrexone is 8 mg for patients weighing 38– 62 kg or 12 mg for patients weighing 62 – 114 kg. Patients whose weight falls outside of these ranges should be dosed at 0.15 mg / kg (43).

Alvimopan

Alvimopan is an orally administered, peripherally acting μ -opioid receptor antagonist that does not cross the blood – brain barrier at clinically relevant dosages (44) and does not reverse analgesia or cause opioid withdrawal symptoms. At the moment, Alvimopan is not approved for treatment of OIC. However, there is already significant literature about its potential in OIC associated with chronic opioid therapy.

In a study of 522 subjects reporting < 3 spontaneous bowel movements (SBMs) per week and a pain treatment with ≥ 30 mg oral morphine equivalent unit / day, were evaluated the efficacy of alvimapan on OIC. (45) Participants were randomized to receive alvimopan, 0.5 mg b.i.d., 1 mg once daily, 1 mg b.i.d., or placebo for 6 weeks (45). There was a significant increase in mean SBM / week over the initial 3 weeks of treatment with all 3 doses of alvimopan tested, as well as improvements in straining, stool consistency, incomplete evacuation, abdominal bloating/discomfort, and decreased appetite, which were sustained over 6 weeks. The most frequent adverse events were abdominal pain, nausea, and diarrhea, occurring more frequently in the higher dosage groups. The alvimopan 0.5 mg b.i.d. dose demonstrated the best benefit-to-risk profile for managing OBD, with a side-effect profile similar to that of placebo (45). There was no evidence of opioid analgesia antagonism.

NKTR-118

NKTR-118 is an oral PEGylated naloxol conjugate that blocks peripheral μ -opioid receptors in the gut. PEGylation of naloxone alters its distribution, reducing central nervous system penetration and metabolism (reduced first-pass effect) while retaining its opioid antagonist properties peripherally (46).

In human pharmacodynamic studies, NKTR-118 normalized morphine-induced delay in orocecal transit (47), while central effects were maintained with uninhibited pupillary constriction.

In a phase 2, placebo-controlled clinical trial of NKTR-118 in OIC patients (< 3 SBM/ week, on a stable opioid dose of 30– 1,000 morphine-equivalent unit / day for ≥ 2 weeks), 208 patients were randomized into three sequential cohorts of 5, 25, or 50 mg for 4 consecutive weeks aft er a 1-week placebo run-in phase. Patients receiving 25 mg or 50 mg (but not 5 mg) NKTR-118 had significantly increased (over baseline) number of SBM during the first week of treatment (primary end point) and over the 28-day treatment period, compared with placebo. There was no evidence of opioid withdrawal, reversal of analgesia, or increase in opioid use at any dose tested. Most frequent side eff ects were abdominal cramping, diarrhea, nausea, and vomiting, which were more frequent in the 50 mg cohort. *TD-1211* TD-1211 is an orally administered, peripherally selective, multivalent inhibitor of the μ - opioid receptor. It has high affinity for human μ - and δ -receptors, and guinea-pig μ -opioid receptors, with > 6,000-fold selectivity for the μ –opioid receptor over non-opioid receptors, ligand-gated ion channels, enzymes, ion channels (including hERG), and transporters. It inhibits loperamide-induced reduction in gastric emptying and attenuation of castor oil-induced diarrhea following acute oral dosing to conscious rats.

3.5 Prucalopride, a prokinetic 5-HT 4 receptor agonist

Prucalopride is a new, selective 5-HT 4 agonist with efficacy in relief of chronic constipation and safety from a cardiovascular perspective. In a phase 2, double-blind, placebo-controlled study 196 patients with OIC were randomized to receive placebo, prucalopride 2 or 4 mg for 4 weeks. The increase from baseline of ≥ 1 spontaneous complete bowel movements (SCBM) per week (weeks 1 - 4, primary end point) was greater in the prucalopride groups (35.9 % (2 mg) and 40.3% (4 mg) than placebo (23.4%), reaching statistical significance in week 1. Prucalopride, 4 mg, significantly improved patient-rated severity of constipation and effectiveness of treatment vs. placebo, and improved Patient Assessment of Constipation - Symptom (PAC-SYM) total scores and Patient Assessment of Constipation-Quality of Life (PAC-QOL) total and satisfaction subscale scores. The most common adverse events were abdominal pain and nausea.

Lubiprostone

Lubiprostone is a chloride channel activator that induces intestinal secretion.

Lubiprostone, in vitro, stimulates chloride secretion that was suppressed by morphine. *In vivo,* instead, s.c. lubiprostone increased fecal wet weight and numbers of pellets expelled in guinea-pig and mouse (48) reduced by Morphine.

Injection of lubiprostone, 30 min after morphine, reversed morphine-induced suppression of fecal wet weight. The data suggest that lubiprostone, bypasses the neurogenic constipating effects of morphine by directly opening chloride channels in the mucosal epithelium (48).

4. Conclusion

The management of patients with OIC is an increasingly relevant problem with the extensive use of opioids for the relief of chronic pain, often associated with benign conditions. Several novel pharmacological approaches are being developed, including assessment of promotility and secreta- gogue agents that have efficacy in chronic idiopathic constipation. Other approaches are directed at the reversal of peripheral opiate effects in the gut while maintaining the desired analgesic efficacy. Several new approaches are promising, including tapentadol, combination of opioids with prolonged release naloxone, NKTR-118, and TD-1211. An evidence-based management approach for OIC will be more feasible after the new generation of drugs is formally and thoroughly studied in large, high-quality clinical trials.

5. References

[1] Verhaak PF, Kerssens JJ, Dekker J et al. Prevalence of chronic benign pain disorder among adults: A review of the literature. Pain 1998; 77 : 231 - 9.

[2] Blyth FM, March LM, Brnabic AJ et al. Chronic pain in Australia: a prevalence study. Pain 2001; 89 : 127 - 34.

[3] Breivik H, Collett B, Ventafridda V et al. Survey of chronic pain in Europe: prevalence, impact on daily life, and treatment. Eur J Pain 2006; 10 : 287 - 333.

[4] Trescot AM, Helm S, Hansen H et al. Opioids in the management of chronic non-cancer pain: an update of American Society of the Interventional Pain Physicians' (ASIPP) Guidelines. Pain Physician 2008; 11 (2 Suppl) : S5 - S62.

[5] Kalso E, Edwards JE, Moore A et al. Opioids in chronic non-cancer pain:systematic review of effi cacy and safety. Pain 2004; 112 : 372 - 80.

[6] Papagallo M. Incidence, prevalence and management of opioid bowel dysfunction. Am J Surg 2001; 182 (November Suppl) : S11 - 8.

[7] Benyamin R, Trescot AM, Datta S et al. Opioid complications and side effects. Pain Physician 2008; 11 (2 Suppl) : S105 - 20.

[8] Pappagallo M. Incidence, prevalence, and management of opioid bowel dysfunction. Am J Surg 2001; 182 (5A Suppl) : 11S - 8S.

[9] Rang HP, Dale MM, Ritter JM. Analgesic drugs. Pharmacology 1999; 13 : 579 - 603.

[10] Kurz A, Sessler DI. Opioid-induced bowel dysfunction: pathophysiology and potential new therapies. Drugs 2003; 63 : 649 - 71.

[11] Stefano GB, Goumon Y, Casares F et al. Endogenous morphine. Trends Neurosci 2000; 23 : 436 - 42.

[12] Bagnol D, Mansour A, Akil H et al. Cellular localization and distribution of the cloned mu and kappa opioid receptors in rat gastrointestinal tract. Neuroscience 1997; 81 : 579 - 91.

[13] McKay JS, Linaker BD, Turnberg LA. Infl uence of opiates on ion transport across rabbit ileal mucosa. Gastroenterology 1981; 80 : 279 - 84.

[14] Fickel J, Bagnol D, Watson SJ et al. Opioid receptor expression in the rat gastrointestinal tract: a quantitative study with comparison to the brain. Brain Res Mol Brain Res 1997; 46 : 1 - 8.

[15] De Schepper HU, Cremonini F, Park MI et al. Opioids and the gut: pharmacology and current clinical experience. Neurogastroenterol Motil 2004; 16 : 383 - 94.

[16] Wood JD, Galligan JJ. Function of opioids in the enteric nervous system. Neurogastroenterol Motil 2004; 16 (Suppl 2) : 17 - 28.

[17] Kress HG. Tapentadol and its two mechanisms of action: is there a new pharmacological class of centrally-acting analgesics on the horizon? Eur J Pain 2010; 14 : 781 - 3.

[18] Chial HJ, Camilleri M, Ferber I et al. Eff ects of venlafaxine, buspirone, and placebo on colonic sensorimotor functions in healthy humans. Clin Gastroenterol Hepatol 2003; 1 : 211 - 8.

[19] Viramontes BE, Malcolm A, Camilleri M et al. Eff ects of an alpha(2)-adrenergic agonist on gastrointestinal transit, colonic motility, and sensation in humans. Am J Physiol Gastroint Liver Physiol 2001; 281 : G1468 - 76.

[20] Camilleri M, Busciglio I, Carlson P et al. Pharmacogenetics of low dose clonidine in irritable bowel syndrome. Neurogastroenterol Motil 2009; 21 : 399 - 410.

[21] Candiotti KA, Gitlin MC. Review of the eff ect of opioid-related side eff ects on the undertreatment of moderate to severe chronic noncancer pain: tapentadol, a step toward a solution? Curr Med Res Opin 2010; 26 : 1677 - 84.

[22] Afilalo M, Etropolski MS, Kuperwasser B et al. Effi cacy and safety of tapentadol extended release compared with oxycodone controlled release for the management of moderate to severe chronic pain related to osteoarthritis of the knee: results of a randomized, double-blind, placebo- and activecontrolled phase 3 study. Clinical Drug Invest 2010; 30 : 489 - 505.

[23] Buynak R, Shapiro DY, Okamoto A et al. Efficacy and safety of tapentadol extended release for the management of chronic low back pain: results of a prospective, randomized, double-blind, placebo- and active-controlled phase III study. Expert Opin Pharmacother 2010; 11 : 1787 - 804.

[24] Meissner W, Schmidt U, Hartmann M e t al. Oral naloxone reverses opioid associated constipation. Pain 2000; 84 : 105 - 9.

[25] Sykes NP. An investigation of the ability of oral naloxone to correct opioid-related constipation in patients with advanced cancer. Palliat Med 1996; 10 : 135 - 44.

[26] Vondrackova D, Leyendecker P, Meissner W et al. Analgesic efficacy and safety of oxycodone in combination with naloxone as prolonged release tablets in patients with moderate to severe chronic pain. J Pain 2008; 9 : 1144 - 54.

[27] Meissner W, Leyendecker P, Mueller-Lissner S et al. A randomised controlled trial with prolonged-release oral oxycodone and naloxone to prevent and reverse opioid-induced constipation. Eur J Pain 2009; 13 : 56 - 64.

[28] Sandner-Kiesling A, Leyendecker P, Hopp M et al. Long-term efficacy and safety of combined prolonged-release oxycodone and naloxone in the management of non-cancer chronic pain. Int J Clin Pract 2010; 64 : 763 - 74.

[29] Webster LR, Brewer R, Wang C et al. Long-term safety and effi cacy of morphine sulfate and naltrexone hydrochloride extended release capsules, a novel formulation containing morphine and sequestered naltrexone, in patients with chronic, moderate to severe pain. J Pain Symptom Manage 2010; 40 : 734 - 46

[30] Foss JF. A review of the potential role of methyl-naltrexone in opioid bowel dysfunction. Am J Surg 2001; 182 (5A Suppl) : 19S - 26S.

[31] Meissner W, Leyendecker P, Meuller-Lissner S, Nad- stawek J, Hopp M, Ruckes C, Wirz S et al.: A random- ised controlled trial with prolonged-release oral oxyco-

done and naloxone to prevent and reverse opioid-induced constipation. Eur J Pain, 2009, 13, 56–64.

[32] Müller-Lissner S, Leyendecker P, Hopp M, Ruckes C, Fleischer W, Reimer K: Oral prolonged release (PR) oxycodone/naloxone combination reduces opioid- induced bowel dysfunction (OIBD) in patients with se- vere chronic pain. Eur J Pain, 2007, 11, abstract 189

[33] De Shepper HU, Cremonini F, Park MI, Camilleri M: Opioids and the gut: pharmacology and current clinical experience. Neurogastroenterol Motil, 2004, 16, 383–394.

[34] Liu M, Wittbrodt E: Low-dose oral naloxone reverses opioid-induced constipation and analgesia. J Pain Symp- tom Manage, 2002, 23, 48–53.

[35] Davis MP, Varga J, Dickerson D, Walsh D, LeGrand SB, Lagman R: Normal-release and controlled-release oxy- codone: pharmacokinetics, pharmacodynamics, and con- troversy. Support Care Cancer, 2003, 11, 84–92.

[36] Yuan CS. Methylnaltrexone mechanisms of action and eff ects on opioid bowel dysfunction and other opioid adverse eff ects. Ann Pharmacother 2007; 41 : 984 - 93.

[37] Yuan CS, Foss JF, O ' Connor M et al. Methylnaltrexone for reversal of constipation due to chronic methadone use: a randomized controlled trial. JAMA 2000; 283 : 367 - 72.

[38] Yuan CS, Foss JF, Osinski J et al. Th e safety and effi cacy of oral methylnaltrexone in preventing morphine-induced delay in oral-cecal transit time. Clin Pharmacol Th er 1997; 61 : 467 - 75.

[39] Yuan CS, Foss JF, O' Connor M et al. Methylnaltrexone prevents morphine- induced delay in oral-cecal transit time without aff ecting analgesia: a double-blind randomized placebo-controlled trial. Clin Pharmacol Ther 1996; 59 : 469 - 75.

[40] Thomas J, Karver S, Cooney GA et al. Methylnaltrexone for opioid-induced constipation in advanced illness. N Engl J Med 2008; 358 : 2332 - 43.

[41] Lang L. Th e food and drug administration approves methylnaltrexone bromide for opioid-induced constipation. Gastroenterology 2008; 135 : 6.

[42] http://www.thomsonhc.com/hcs/librarian/MICROMEDEX: Physician's Desk Reference: methylnaltrexone.

[43] Schmidt WK. Alvimopan (ADL 8-298) is a novel peripheral opioid antagonist. Am J Surg 2001; 182 : 27S - 38S.

[44] Webster L, Jansen JP, Peppin J et al. Alvimopan, a peripherally acting mu-opioid receptor (PAM-OR) antagonist for the treatment of opioid induced bowel dysfunction: results from a randomized, double-blind, placebo-controlled, dose-fi nding study in subjects taking opioids for chronic non-cancer pain. Pain 2008; 137 : 428 - 40.

[45] Eldon MA, Song D, Neumann TA et al. Oral NKTR-118 (oral PEGnaloxol), a PEGylated derivative of naloxone; demonstration of selective peripheral opioid antagonism aft er oral administration in preclinical models. American Academy of Pain Management 18th Annual Clinical Mtg., Las Vegas, NV, 27 - 30 September 2007, poster 28.

[46] Neumann TA, van Paaschen H, Marcantonio A et al. Clinical investigation of oral NKTR-118 as a selective oral peripheral opioid antagonist. 18th Annual Clinical Mtg. of the American Academy of Pain Management, Las Vegas, NV, Sept. 27-30, 2007, abstract 27.

[47] Fei G, Raehal K, Liu S et al. Lubiprostone reverses the inhibitory action of morphine on intestinal secretion in guinea pig and mouse. J Pharmacol Exp Th er 2010; 334 : 333 - 40.

7

Drugs in Development for Opioid-Induced Constipation

Kelly S. Sprawls, Egilius L.H. Spierings and Dustin Tran
MedVadis Research Corporation
USA

1. Introduction

Opioid-induced bowel dysfunction (OIBD) is a collective term used to describe the gastrointestinal side effects of long-term opioid therapy in chronic pain patients. Constipation, nausea, vomiting, bloating, abdominal pain, and gastric reflux are among the most common gastrointestinal adverse effects. Within opioid-induced bowel dysfunction, a more specific subset exists, opioid-induced constipation, characterized by infrequent stools, straining, hard, dry stools, and incomplete evacuation. In these patients, the constipation can be so severe that they are willing to compromise their pain management by reducing their opioid analgesic dose, switch to a less potent opioid with inadequate pain relief, or completely discontinue their opioid medication all together. It is evident that opioid-induced constipation remains a significant barrier to achieving optimal pain management and represents a large unmet medical NEED.

Opioids induce gastrointestinal side effects indirectly through an effect on the central nervous system and directly through an effect on the gastrointestinal tract. Related to the indirect effect, it has been shown that intrathecal administration of opioids decreases gastrointestinal motility and intestinal secretion (Anderson, 2007). The direct effect is mediated through mu-opioid receptors in the neuronal plexi, located between the longitudinal and circular muscle layers (myenteric plexus) and within the submucosa (submucosal plexus). Within the myenteric plexus, the opioids induce relaxation of the longitudinal smooth-muscle layer and increase tonicity in the circular smooth-muscle layer. These effects are thought to be mediated through inhibition of acetylcholine release and inhibition of vasoactive intestinal peptide and nitric oxide release, respectively. The result of this differential effect on the longitudinal and circular intestinal smooth muscles is an increase in segmental contraction and a decrease in peristaltic activity.

Normal peristalsis in the small bowel occurs every 90 minutes in order to move the luminal contents from the duodenum to the ileum. Mass movements in the large bowel occurs less often, one to three times per day, sweeping its contents over longer distances. As a result of the reduced peristalic activity, the transit time is significantly prolonged. The food stays in the stomach longer and the stool resides in the small and large bowel. The former causes gastric distension, resulting in nausea and gastric reflux, and the latter contributes to the constipation by allowing more time for fluid absorption, a predominant function of the large bowel in particular. A decrease in bowel-movement frequency is the primary symptom of constipation, with secondary symptoms being hard, dry stool, the need for straining with bowel movements, and a sense of incomplete evacuation. Tertiary symptoms are abdominal bloating/distension, discomfort, and pain from stool or gas, borborygmi, flatulence, and dyspnea from interference of the abdominal stool and gas content with diaphragmatic contraction aiding inspiration. Aside from these physiologic effects exuded by the opioid analgesics themselves, the lifestyle of patients in chronic pain typically intensifies their condition. Chronic pain patients are often inactive and deconditioned. They are more likely to be overweight, have a poor diet, and get little to no exercise, exacerbating their constipation.

2. Prevalence

In 2010, it was estimated that approximately 250 million prescriptions were written for opioids in the United States (IMS Health 2010) and many studies indicate that a high percentage of patients receiving opioids experience gastrointestinal side effects. A systematic review was performed of 11 randomized, double-blind, placebo-controlled studies of oral opioids in the treatment of chronic non-cancer pain, given for periods ranging from 4 days to 8 weeks (Kalso et al., 2004). The opioids were morphine in five studies, morphine or methadone in one study, and oxycodone in four studies; all studies used inactive placebo except two in which benztropine was given as active placebo. Of the 1,025 subjects randomized, 674 subjects completed the study they were in and 698 subjects were evaluable. Adverse events and lack of efficacy were the most frequent reasons for discontinuation during both opioid and placebo treatment. The mean final daily doses of the oral opioids varied from 30 to 120 mg for morphine, 20 to 45 mg for oxycodone (30 to 68.5 mg morphine equivalents), and 15 mg for methadone (45 mg morphine equivalents).

Constipation was the most common adverse event in the opioid-treated subjects, reported by 41% of the subjects in comparison to 11% of those treated with placebo, followed by nausea (32% *versus* 12%). The actual occurrence of constipation with oral opioid treatment in the range of 30 to 120 mg morphine equivalents per day is probably higher. The enriched nature of the studies excluded subjects from randomization who did not tolerate the medication or who did not find it effective in relieving their pain. The subjects who were not randomized because of the latter reason would also have discontinued the medication in practice; however, the subjects who were not randomized because of tolerability reasons would possibly have continued the treatment if the adverse event was constipation and this was effectively treated.

3. Available treatments

In 2008, the Food and Drug Administration approved a peripherally-acting mu-opioid-receptor antagonist (PAMORA), subcutaneous methylnaltrexone (Relistor®), for the treatment of opioid-induced constipation in patients with advanced illness who are receiving palliative care when response to traditional laxative therapy has been inadequate. Another peripherally-acting mu-opioid-receptor antagonist, alvimopan, was being studied as well but cardiovascular safety concerns, consisting of an increased risk of myocardial infarction, halted drug development. However, the Food and Drug Administration approved the medication in 2008 with a Risk Evaluation and Mitigation Strategy (REMS) for the indication of accelerating the time to upper and lower gastrointestinal recovery, following partial small- or large-bowel resection with primary anastomosis. The Risk

Evaluation and Mitigation Strategy restricts the use of the medication to short-term (15 doses) treatment in hospitalized patients and only in hospitals that have registered with the program and have met all the requirements.

Lubiprostone and tegaserod are Food and Drug Administration approved for the treatment of chronic idiopathic constipation in adults and can, of course, be used off label for this condition as well. Lubiprostone is an activator of the ClC-2 chloride channel, increasing water secretion in the lumen of the gastrointestinal tract, and tegaserod is a non-selective serotonin-4-receptor agonist. However, in 2007, upon request from the Food and Drug Administration, alleging increased risk of cardiovascular and cerebrovascular events, Novartis withdrew tegaserod from the market. Prior to its withdrawal, tegaserod was being studied for opioid-induced constipation. A prokinetic medication could be used as well, although not approved by the Food and Drug Administration for (opioid-induced) constipation, such as cisapride, a non-selective serotonin-4-receptor agonist, domperidone, a peripherally-acting dopamine-receptor antagonist, or metoclopramide, a dopamine-2-receptor antagonist and mixed serotonin-3-receptor antagonist/serotonin-4-receptor agonist. However, cisapride was withdrawn from the market because of long QT syndrome predisposing to arrhythmias, domperidone is not on the market in the United States, and the long-term, daily use of metoclopramide is not recommended because of potential extrapyramidal side effects, particularly tardive dyskinesia. Misoprostol, a synthetic prostaglandin E1 analogue, approved by the Food and Drug Administration for the prevention of gastric ulcers caused by the use of non-steroidal anti-inflammatory drugs (NSAIDs), also increases colonic transit and can be used off label as well.

Another strategy that is used to treat opioid-induced constipation is to switch to an opioid that, in general, causes less constipation as a side effect. From a constipation perspective and according to our experience, morphine, codeine, and hydrocodone tend to be worse and, for example, oxycodone and fentanyl better. Opioids that produce analgesia through other mechanisms, such as tramadol and tapentadol, which apart from being mu-opioid-receptor agonists also inhibit the presynaptic uptake of noradrenaline, tend to cause less constipation.

Over the counter constipation products in general can also be used for opioid-induced constipation, such as bulking agents (cellulose, psyllium), stool softeners (docusate), osmotic agents (lactulose, sorbitol, magnesium citrate, polyethylene glycol), and laxatives (senna, bisacodyl). Although traditional laxatives have proved efficacious at inducing bowel movments, they are a temporary, quick fix and frequently induce undesired side effects. For many patients a successful bowel movement requires a cumbersome combination of stool softeners, bowel stimulants, and osmotic agents. The unpredictable nature of stimulant laxatives are unappealing for patients as well. Aggressive laxative use does not come without the risk of serious side effects, including metabolic abnormalities, and the long term safety and relief of abdominal symptoms has yet to be revealed. One exception is Miralax (polyethylene glycol) which demonstrated sustained efficacy in long-term studies. Furthermore, traditional laxatives are not specifically approved by the Food and Drug Administration (FDA) for opioid-induced constipation.

4. Drug development

Given the paucity of FDA-approved medications and the sub-optimal efficacy of over the counter options for the treatment of opioid-induced constipation, a new drug class, peripherally-acting mu-opioid receptor antagonists (PAMORAs), has evolved that directly targets the mechanism of opioid-induced constipation. The first two drugs to enter the market were subcutanous methylnaltrexone (Relistor®) in April 2008 and an oral formulation of alvimopan (Entereg®) in May 2008. However, both drugs were FDA-approved in a specific sub-population, palliative care patients and post-surgical patients, respectively. Thus, the treatment for the general population with opioid-induced constipation reamined limited. Since 2008, several pharmaceutical companies have developed peripherally-acting mu-opioid receptor antagonists that are now undergoing various phases of clinical studies with the specific indication of opioid-induced constipation in chronic pain patients.

Peripherally-acting mu opioid-receptor antagonists are an improvement to the traditional non-specific opioid-antagonists, naloxone and naltrexone. The novelty behind the new class resides with its restricted activity to the peripheral mu-opioid receptors in the enteric system and increased specificity to the mu-receptors versus the kappa- and delta-receptors. As a result, the constipating effects of opioids on gastrointestinal function and motility are inhibited without crossing the blood-brain barrier and reversing the central analgesic effects of opioids.

Amoung the drugs currently being developed, the oral formulation is the most popular. While subcutaneous methylnaltrexone (Relistor) has already been approved by the Food and Drug Administration, clinical studies with the oral formulation are underway. Other oral, peripherally-acting mu-opioid receptor antagonists in development for opioid-induced constipation are ADL5945 (Adolor), ALKS37 (Alkermes), NKTR-118 (AstraZeneca), S-297995 (Shionogi), and TD-1211 (Theravance). Lubiprostone, already FDA-approved for other types of constipation, is undergoing development for opioid-induced constipation as well. Medications that are in development for chronic constipation and may ultimately also be developed for opioid-induced constipation are the selective serotonin-4-receptor agonist, prucalopride (Johnson & Johnson), and the guanylate-cyclase C-receptor agonists, linaclotide (Ironwood) and plecanatide (Synergy).

4.1 Methylnaltrexone

Methylnaltrexone is a quaternary derivative of naltrexone, synthesized by adding a methyl group to the nitrogen atom of the molecule. Quaternary opioid antagonists are constructed to have more polarity and, therefore, less lipid solubility than their parent compounds. The reduced ability to penetrate the blood-brain barrier allows the medications to block opioid-induced constipation peripherally, without antagonizing the centrally-mediated opioid analgesia or causing central opioid withdrawal.

Methylnaltrexone was initially tested in an intravenous formulation. A laxation response was seen in 11 subjects with methadone-induced constipation who were treated with methylnaltrexone IV, compared to no laxation response in the 11 subjects in the placebo group ($P<0.001$)[2]. Along with the 100% response rate in the methylnaltrexone recipients, no central opioid withdrawal was observed and no significant adverse events were reported. At the same time, the oral-cecal transit time was decreased by 77.7 minutes from baseline in the methylnaltrexone group, while only by 1.4 minutes in the placebo group ($p<0.001$). Subsequently, subcutaneous administration was studied, potentially enlarging the target population for this treatment.

In a double-blind, randomized, placebo-controlled study in healthy volunteers, oral-cecal transit time was significantly reduced after 0.3 mg/kg subcutaneous methylnaltrexone plus morphine, compared with placebo plus morphine (P<0.05) ((Yuan et al, 2002). As an intervention for opioid-induced constipation in advanced illness, 0.15 mg/kg subcutaneous methylnaltrexone caused a laxation response within 4 hours in 48% of 62 subjects in the methylnaltrexone group, compared to 15% of the 71 subjects in the placebo group (p<0.001). Fifty two percent of the subjects had laxation without the use of a rescue laxative within 4 hours after two or more of the first four doses, as compared to 8% in the placebo group (P<0.001) ((Thomas et al, 2008). The treatment did not affect centrally-mediated analgesia and did not precipitate opioid withdrawal. Abdominal pain and flatulence were the most common adverse events.

A similar study in opioid-induced constipation in advanced illness used a single subcutaneous injection of methylnaltrexone, 0.15 mg/kg or 0.3 mg/kg, or placebo (Slatkin et al, 2009). Sixty two percent and 58% of the subjects treated with methylnaltrexone 0.15 mg/kg and 0.3 mg/kg, respectively, had a laxation response within 4 hours, compared to 14% of the subjects in the placebo group (P<0.0001; each dose *versus* placebo). Adverse events were slightly more common in the subjects treated with 0.15 mg/kg than in those treated with 0.3 mg/kg, particularly abdominal pain, flatulence, nausea, and dizziness. Due to a comparable efficacy profile, the results suggest the lower dose, 0.15 mg/kg, to be most optimal.

Methylnaltrexone in a dose of 12 mg subcutaneous was given once daily or every other day for 28 days in a randomized, double-blind, placebo-controlled study, which involved a total of 469 subjects with opioid-induced constipation (Slatkin et al, 2009). Compared to placebo, the medication given once daily significantly improved rectal symptoms (P<0.05), stool symptoms (P<0.001), and global constipation scores (P<0.001), while given every other day significantly improved stool symptoms (P<0.05) and global constipation scores (P<0.05). The changes from baseline in abdominal symptoms and pain scores between the two methylnaltrexone groups and placebo were not significant.

Although the intravenous and subcutaneous formulations produced promising results, they are impractical for the general population. An intravenous administration can only be administered under the supervision of health care professionals, and while the subcutaneous injections are more safe and convenient, they either require self-administration or frequent assistance. An oral formulation is the most favorable as a pill is generally more convenient and affordable. Fortunately, phase 3 studies have commenced, assessing the safety and efficacy of oral methylnaltrexone for opioid-induced constipation in chronic pain patients.

4.2 ADL5945

ADL5945 is an oral peripherally-acting mu-opioid-receptor antagonist in development by Adolor with two randomized, double-blind, placebo-controlled studies recently completed in subjects with chronic non-cancer pain and opioid-induced constipation. In the first study, two doses of ADL5945 (0.10 mg and 0.25 mg) were given twice daily *versus* placebo to 130 subjects (43 per treatment arm) over 4 weeks. The second study was of similar design, with the exception that only one dose of ADL5945 (0.25 mg) was given and only once daily *versus* placebo to 80 patients (40 per treatment arm). The primary endpoint in both studies was the change from baseline in the mean number of spontaneous bowel movements per week over the 4-week treatment period. The results demonstrated a statistically significant and clinically relevant effect of the 0.25 mg dose in particular, without tolerability issues and evidence of central opioid withdrawal or reversal of opioid analgesia. Adolor's backup compound for opioid-induced constipation is the peripherally-acting mu-opioid-receptor antagonist, ADL7745, which recently successfully completed preclinical studies.

4.3 ALKS37

ALKS 37 (RDC-1036) is an oral peripherally-acting mu-opioid-receptor antagonist in development by Alkermes for the treatment of opioid-induced constipation, with a randomized, double-blind, placebo-controlled, multi-dose study recently completed (Alkermes website, 2011). The study treated opioid-induced constipation in subjects with chronic non-cancer pain with doses of 1 to 100 mg taken once daily. Subjects were eligible to participate in the study if they were taking opioid analgesics at doses of 30 mg or more morphine equivalents per day and had fewer than three spontaneous bowel movements per week.

The primary endpoint was a change from baseline in the average number of spontaneous bowel movements per week. A clear dose-response relationship was demonstrated with a statistically significant increase in the average number of spontaneous bowel movements per week in the subjects receiving 100 mg of the medication once daily, compared to those receiving placebo (4.5 *versus* 0.7) ($p = 0.006$). The results also demonstrated a statistically significant increase in the average number of complete spontaneous bowel movements per week, compared to subjects receiving placebo (3.5 *versus* 0.8) ($p = 0.007$). Overall, ALKS 37 was well tolerated and the most commonly reported adverse events were gastrointestinal in nature, including abdominal pain (25%) and diarrhea (22%), mostly occurring in the higher and most effective doses (30 mg and 100 mg). There was no indication of reversal of opioid analgesia, that is, there was no increase in average daily pain score or opioid use (Alkermes Press Release, 2011).

4.4 NKTR-118

NKTR-118, also known as PEG-naloxol, is a combination of naloxol, a derivative of the opioid antagonist, naloxone, and a polyethylene glycol moiety. The purpose of the PEGylation is twofold, that is: 1. altering its metabolism, thereby reducing the first-pass effect and increasing its bioavailability, and 2. modifying its distribution to reduce penetration into the central nervous system. A randomized, double-blind, placebo-controlled, multiple-dose study was performed, evaluating the safety and efficacy of NKTR-118 in subjects with opioid-induced constipation (Webster, L., 2009). Eligible subjects were defined as having opioid-induced constipation with fewer than three spontaneous bowel movements per week and on a stable analgesic opioid regimen of 30 mg to 1000 mg morphine equivalents per day for a minimum of 2 weeks. A total of 208 subjects were randomized to NKTR-118 or placebo in three sequential cohorts. The first week they received a once daily dose of single-blind placebo, followed by 4 weeks of NKTR-118 once daily in doses of 5, 25, or 50 mg, or placebo.

The primary endpoint was achieved in both the 25-mg and 50-mg treatment groups, with a significant increase in the mean number of spontaneous bowel movements per week over the first week. Subjects receiving 25 mg NKTR-118 had an average of 5.0 spontaneous bowel movements during the first week (1.4 at baseline) *versus* 3.1 in the placebo group (1.2 at baseline)($p = 0.002$). Subjects receiving 50 mg NKTR-118 had an average of 6.0 spontaneous bowel movements during the first week (1.6 at baseline) *versus* 3.3 in the placebo group (1.3 at baseline)($p = 0.0001$). The increase in bowel movements was sustained at a statistically significant level throughout the 4 weeks in both dose groups ($p = 0.002$ and $p<0.0001$, respectively). The medication was well tolerated and adverse events were dose-dependent, occurring most frequently in the 50-mg group, and were primarily gastrointestinal in nature, particularly abdominal pain, cramps, diarrhea, and nausea. The majority of the adverse events were rated as mild or moderate in intensity. Reversal of opioid analgesia was not observed in the study, as measured by numerical pain rating and opioid requirement.

4.5 S-297995

Shionogi has developed an oral peripherally-acting mu-opioid-receptor antagonist, S-297995. Initially, it was designed to alleviate a spectrum of opioid-induced side effects (constipation, nausea, and vomiting) but the more recent studies have focused primarily on its effects on opioid-induced constipation. S-297995 may prove more favorable than existing treatments, given its efficacy at lower doses in alleviating not just opioid-induced constipation but also nausea and vomiting (Shionogi website, 2011).

In 2011, a randomized, double-blind, placebo-controlled, single-ascending dose study was completed to evaluate the safety and efficacy of S-297995 in opioid-induced constipation. Subjects were eligible to participate in the study if they had chronic pain requiring 90 mg or more morphine equivalents daily for a minimum of 3 months, opioid-induced constipation, and physical opioid dependence. Seventy five subjects were randomized to one of six S-297995 cohorts (0.01 mg, 0.03 mg, 0.1 mg, 0.3 mg, 1.0 mg, or 3.0 mg). Preliminary results demonstrate a statistically significant and dose-dependent increase from baseline in the number of spontaneous bowel movements at 24 hours post-dose, starting at doses of 0.3 mg ($p = 0.0011$ in the 0.3-mg group and $p<0.001$ in both the 1.0-mg and 3.0-mg groups). The medication was generally well tolerated with predominantly mild or moderate gastrointestinal adverse events. There was no evidence of central opioid withdrawal and there was no impact on the analgesic effect of the opioids or a change in pupil size (Shionogi Annual Report, 2011).

4.6 TD-1211

TD-1211 is a multivalent compound designed by Theravance to block the effects of opioids on the gastrointestinal mu-opioid receptors, without mitigating their central analgesic properties. In preclinical studies, the medication demonstrated oral bioavailability with no evidence of activity in the central nervous system. A randomized, double-blind, placebo-controlled, dose-escalation study assessed the efficacy and safety of the medication in subjects with non-cancer pain and opioid-induced constipation (Theravance Press Release, 2011). The latter was defined as fewer than five spontaneous bowel movements during a 2-week baseline period and at least one additional symptom of constipation. A total of 70 subjects were randomized to receive oral 0.25, 0.75, 2.0, 5.0, and 10.0 mg doses of TD 1211 daily, or placebo.

The primary endpoint was the change from baseline in the average spontaneous bowel movements per week over the 2-week treatment period. Proof of efficacy was achieved in a dose-dependent fashion, specifically with the 5 and 10 mg doses. In the subjects who received the 5 mg dose, the mean number of spontaneous bowel movements increased by 3.2 (from 1.1 at baseline to 4.3 over the 2-week treatment period; confidence interval: 1.5-5.0). Similarly, in the subjects who received the 10 mg dose, the mean number of spontaneous bowel movements increased by 4.9 (from 1.4 at baseline to 6.3 over the 2-week treatment period; confidence interval: 3.1-6.7). However, in the placebo-treated group, the increase in the mean number of spontaneous bowel movements was not statistically significant (from 1.7 at baseline to 3.3 over the 2-week treatment period; confidence interval: 0.6-2.5).

Regarding the median time to first spontaneous bowel movement after the first dose of TD-1211, a dose-dependent reduction was observed in the subjects receiving the 5 and 10 mg doses, with the time reduced to 8.6 and 3.6 hours, respectively, *versus* 28.7 hours in the placebo group. Overall, TD-1211 was well tolerated with the majority of the gastrointestinal adverse events mild or moderate in intensity, occurring early in treatment and resolving within days. There was no evidence of central opioid withdrawal with the medication or reversal of opioid analgesia.

4.7 Lubiprostone

Lubiprostone is an activator of the CIC-2 chloride channel, increasing water secretion in the lumen of the gastrointestinal tract, approved by the Food and Drug Administration for the treatment of chronic constipation and constipation-predominant irritable bowel syndrome (IBS). It is in development for opioid-induced constipation and two randomized, double-blind, placebo-controlled studies with this indication have been completed (Sucampo website, 2009). The two studies are identical phase 3 trials in which a total of 875 subjects with opioid-induced bowel dysfunction were randomized to 12-week treatment with lubiprostone, 24 mcg twice daily. The subjects were taking opioid medications for chronic non-cancer pain, including fentanyl, methadone, morphine, and oxycodone, for at least 30 days prior to screening and continued to take these medications for the duration of the study. During the 2-week baseline period before randomization, they were required to have fewer than three spontaneous bowel movements per week. The overall adverse-event rate for the combined studies was 54.9% for lubiprostone and 51.6% for placebo, with nausea being most common (15.0% *versus* 7.5%), followed by diarrhea (8.5% *versus* 3.7%).

The primary endpoint of the studies was the change from baseline in the frequency of spontaneous bowel movements at week 8 of treatment, which was met in one of the studies (OBD0631) but not in the other (OBD0632). The change from baseline in the frequency of spontaneous bowel movements in the first study was from 1.42 to 4.54 for lubiprostone and from 1.46 to 3.81 for placebo; in the second study, these changes were from 1.60 to 4.10 for lubiprostone and from 1.60 to 3.95 for placebo. An interesting post-hoc sub-analysis revealed that subjects taking methadone and randomized to lubiprostone experienced a lower increase in the frequency of spontaneous bowel movements than lubiprostone-treated subjects on other opioids. Methadone was subsequently found to interfere with the mode of action of lubiprostone at the level of the CIC-2 chloride channel. A third randomized, double-blind, placebo-controlled study with the exclusion of methadone users is currently being conducted.

5. Conclusion

Opioid-induced gastrointestinal dysfunction results predominantly from the effect of opioids on the mu-opioid receptors in the gastrointestinal tract. Constipation and nausea are its most common symptoms, probably occurring in at least half of the patients treated with oral opioids. The constipation in particular is not an uncommon reason for patients to discontinue the medication or to take it at a dose that is much lower than required for adequate pain relief. In addition, it can further decrease the quality of life in patients whose quality of life is generally already significantly impaired by chronic pain. With the exception of subcutaneous methylnaltrexone for a subset of patients, there are no medications on the market for the general population with opioid-induced constipation. Prospective treatments are in developement and will undoubtedly obtain marketing approval from the Food and Drug Administration within the next several years. With the emergence of these novel medications that specifically target the pathophysiology of OIC, there is hope for patients who suffer not only from chronic pain but the adverse effects of their opioid pain medication.

6. Acknowledgements

I would like to thank Dr. Spierings for his support and guidance while writing this manuscript.

7. References

Adolor Clinical Pipeline. n.d. *Website*. September 2011, Available from: <http://www.adolor.com/research/index1.asp?page=r-d-pipeline>

Adolor website. n.d. Opioid-Induced Constipation Development Program. *Website*. September 2011, Available from: <http://www.adolor.com/research/index.asp?page=obd-clinical-development-program>

Alkermes Presents Phase 2 Data of ALKS 37 in Late-Breaking Oral Session at Digestive Disease Week Meeting. n.d. In: *Press Release*, September 2011. Available from: <http://investor.alkermes.com/phoenix.zhtml?c=92211&p=irol-newsArticle&ID=1561623&highlight=>

Alkermes website. n.d. Our Products. *Website*. September 2011, Available from: <http://www.alkermes.com/our-products/in-development.aspx>

Anderson, V. & Burchiel, K as cited in Ruan, Xiulu. (2007). Drug-Related Side Effects of Long Term Intrathecal Morphine Thaerpy. Pain Physician, Vol. 10, (March 2007), pp. 357-365.

IMS Health (2010). September 2011. Available from: <http://www.imshealth.com/deployedfiles/ims/Global/Content/Corporate/Press%20Room/Top-line%20Market%20Data/2010%20Top-line%20Market%20Data/2010_Top_Therapeutic_Classes_by_RX.pdf>

Iyer, S., Randazzo, B. & Tzanis, E. (2011). Effect of subcutaneous methylnaltrexone on patient-reported constipation symptoms. *Value in Health*, Vol. 14, No. 1, (January 2011), pp. 177-183.

Kalso, E., Edwards, J. & Moore, R. (2004). Opioids in chronic non-cancer pain: systematic review of efficacy and safety. *Pain*, Vol. 112, No. 3, (December 2004), pp. 372-380.

Research and Development. n.d. *Shionogi website*, September 2011. Available from: <http://www.shionogi.co.jp/ir_en/explanatory/pdf/e_p110310.pdf>

Shionogi Annual Report 2011. n.d. *Shionogi website*, September 2011. Available from: <http://www.shionogi.co.jp/ir_en/report/pdf_11/business11.pdf>

Slatkin, N., Thomas, J. & Lipman, A. (2009). Methylnaltrexone for Treatment of Opioid-Induced Constipation in Advanced Illness Patients. J. Support Oncol, Vol. 7, No. 1, (January 2009), pp. 39-46.

Sucampo website. n.d. *Website*. July 2009, Available from: <http://investor.sucampo.com>

Theravance Announces Positive Results from Phase 1 and Phase 2 Clinical Studies with TD-1211 in Development for Opioid-Induced Constipation. n.d. *Press Release*, September 2011. Available from: <http://files.shareholder.com/downloads/THERA/1186849209x0x411447/9eac04a8-c982-4ef5-a92d-ff3520f44ccd/PUMA_TD1211.pdf>

Thomas, J., Karver, S. & Cooney, G. (2008). Methylnaltrexone for Opioid-Induced Constipation in Advanced Illness. NEJM, Vol. 358, No. 22, (May 2008), pp. 2332-2343.

Webster, L. (2009) NKTR-118 Significantly Reverses Opioid-Induced Constipation: *Poster, 20th AAPM Annual Clinical Meeting*, September 2011, Available from: <http://nektar.com/pdf/pipeline/NKTR-118/Nektar_poster118AAPM.pdf>

Yuan, C., Foss, J. & O'Conner, M. (2000). Methylnaltrexone for Reversal of Constipation Due to Chronic Methadone Use: A Randomized Controlled Trial. *JAMA*,Vol. 283, No.3, (January 2000), pp. 367-372.

Yuan, C., Wei, G. & Foss, J. (2002). Effects of Subcutaneous Methylnaltrexone on Morphine-Induced Peripherally Mediated Side Effects: A Double-Blind Randomized Placebo-Controlled Trial. JPET, Vol.300, No. 1, (January 2002), pp. 118-123.

8

Constipation Treatment in Neurological Disorders

Gallelli Luca, Pirritano Domenico,
Palleria Caterina and De Sarro Giovambattista
*School of Medicine, University of Catanzaro,
Italy*

1. Introduction

Bowel dysfunction is common in patients with neurological diseases. Its prevalence ranges from 30% to 60% in patients with cerebrovascular diseases and new-onset constipation occurs in 55% of patients after a stroke (Su et al., 2009; Harari et al., 2004; Robain et al., 2002; Bracci et al., 2007). In Multiple Sclerosis (MS) constipation is a frequent bowel symptom and it has been observed in up to 73% of patients (Crayton et al., 2004; Gulick et al., 2011; Wiesel et al., 2000). In Parkinson's disease (PD) constipation is one of the most frequent non-motor features, believed to occur in over 50% of patients (Wood et al., 2010; Pfeiffer et al., 2003; Wolters et al., 2009). Disorders of the anorectal sphincters consist of incontinence or difficulty in expelling faeces. Constipation is almost always associated with slowed bowel transit. It may be due to sphincter incoordination in relation to the detrusor mechanism or to detrusor weakness causing loss of propulsive force (Swash et al., 2001). Constipation may have a significant impact on quality of life and would restrict patient's social activities, increasing levels of anxiety and depression, so that symptoms' management is critically important (Ng et al., 2005). This review describes the possible pathogenesis of constipation in neurological disorders, pharmacological therapies available for constipation and management approaches that may increase the likelihood of satisfactory treatment outcomes.

2. Constipation in stroke

Constipation is defined as two or fewer bowel movements per week, the need to manipulate the rectum digitally to facilitate defecation all or most of the time, and/or use of laxatives, enemas or suppositories more than once a week (Hinds et al., 1990). Medical complications after acute stroke are common, ranging from 28% to 96% (Hong et al., 2008). Bowel dysfunction are the most frequent gastrointestinal complaints with a negative impact on patients' quality of life, restricting their social activities (Bracci et al., 2007; Su et al., 2009). The prevalence of constipation after stroke varies from 30% to 60% (Harari et al., 2004). New-onset constipation is seen in 55% of patients within a month after first stroke, strongly relating to disability. Its development may predict a poor outcome at 12 weeks in patients with moderately severe stroke (Su et al., 2009).

New onset constipation occurs in 30% of hemiplegic patients and has no relationship with the hemispheric side or with the severity of stroke even if a trend of reduced risk of constipation is described in patients with ischemic event and less widespread lesion (Bracci et al., 2007). Risk factors for constipation among stroke patients include use of a number of different drugs, dehydration, older age and immobility (Bracci et al., 2007; Su et al., 2009; Kumar et al., 2010). For the elderly, acute hospitalization is at higher risk to develop constipation than in other age groups (Cardin et al., 2010). The highest risk of new-onset constipation occurs on one week after stroke, so that early intervention may prevent the development of bowel dysfunction (Su et al., 2009). Treatment with nitrates and antithrombotics represents an independent risk factor for developing chronic constipation. Nitrates may cause constipation due to the inhibitory role in gut motility secondary to the release of nitric oxide. Antithrombotic drugs, such as acetyl salicylic acid (ASA), indobufen and ticlopidine, have been reported to be associated with bowel dysfunction. ASA and NSAID are more frequently associated with constipation probably via inhibition of the propulsive activity by preventing the release of prostaglandins. Indobufen and ticlopidine are usually associated with diarrhea. No significant association has been described between new onset constipation and ACE inhibitors or anticoagulants (Bracci et al., 2007). Anticholinergic drugs, such as antipsychotics, tricyclic antidepressants or oxybutynin, significantly increase the risk of faecal incontinence in patients with stroke, decreasing gut motility and causing constipation with overflow incontinence (Kumar et al., 2010). The use of diuretics such as mannitol or furosemide is associated with new-onset constipation (Su et al., 2009).

Bed rest and immobility contribute to constipation onset. Hypovolemia, as a result of dysphagia and/or impaired thirst mechanisms, is another risk factor. Between 37% and 78% of patients with stroke develop dysphagia, with a restriction of oral intake of dietary fibre and a high risk of undernutrition and dehydration (Ullman et al., 1996; Kumar et al., 2010; Su et al., 2009).

It is well known that the central nervous system (CNS) takes part in the control of visceral functions and its damage can lead to gastrointestinal impairment (Bracci et al., 2007). Lesions affecting the pontine defecatory centre may disrupt the sequencing of sympatical and parasympathical components of defecation, and impair the coordination of the peristaltic wave and the relaxation of the pelvic floor and external sphincter (Ullman et al., 1996). Constipation could be a clinical manifestation of spinal cord stroke as a consequence of pelvic autonomic dysfunction (Sakakibara et al., 2008).

3. Constipation in MS

Constipation may represent an early symptom of MS and large bowel impairment can precede the onset of MS by many years (Lawthom et al., 2003; Chellingsworth et al., 2003). Bowel dysfunctions are multifactorial and include neurological impairment, behavioural problems, inappropriate toilet facilities, side effects of drugs or coexistent disorders. A multidisciplinary approach is the best way to deal with this symptom. Bowel symptoms should be carefully treated because sometimes helping constipation can precipitate faecal incontinence. Certain patients would prefer to remain constipated if incontinence is thereby avoided (Wiesel et al., 2001). Gastrointestinal symptoms are common in patients with MS and are much more frequent than in the general population (Wiesel et al., 2001). The prevalence of constipation, alone or in association with faecal incontinence, ranges between 35% to 73%, depending on definitions and selection (Crayton et al., 2004; Gulick et al., 2011; Wiesel et al., 2000; Bakke et al., 1996). There is no difference between male and female patients regarding constipation frequency that presents a strong correlation with disability and disease duration (Hinds et al., 1990). Bladder and bowel dysfunctions have a significant role in psychosocial disability of MS patients, affecting quality of life (Wiesel et al., 2001).

Pathophysiology of constipation in MS is poorly understood. Central nervous system lesions, related to the disease process, may be responsible in some cases, affecting the extrinsic neurological control of gut and sphincter function. Autonomic nervous system impairment, specifically involving parasympathetic pathways, or some systemic mechanism not well known, similar to that which causes fatigue in MS, have been proposed (Fowler et al., 1997; De Seze et al., 2001; Guinet et al., 2011). Some authors have suggested a cerebral involvement or a motor spinal pathways failure as a cause of constipation in MS (Haldeman et al., 1982; Mathers et al., 1990). Abnormalities of colonic activity and prolonged colonic transit time have been demonstrated in some patients, and difficult defecation due to failure to relax the pelvic floor muscles has been found in others (Mark et al., 1999). Whether pelvic floor incoordination shown in some patients with MS should be regarded as a behavioural phenomenon, as in non-neurological constipation, or as related to the MS is yet unknown (Wiesel et al., 2000). Some authors associated large bowel dysfunction to demyelinating lesions of the conus medullaris, even if the role of more proximal lesions cannot be ruled out (Taylor et al., 1984). Other features connected to MS, compromising pelvic floor function and visceral motility, may contribute to constipation: muscle weakness, fatigue, spasticity and poor mobility. Also some medications, commonly used to manage different MS symptoms, such as anticholinergics, antidepressants, opiates and muscle relaxants, can affect bowel function (Wiesel et al., 2001; Fowler et al., 1997; Nordenbo et al., 1996; Gill et al., 1994). Finally, psychological factors or behavioural problems may also affect toileting (Wiesel et al., 2000).

4. Constipation in spinal cord injury

Bowel dysfunction is one of the major sequelae of spinal cord injury (SCI), with a severe impact on long-term quality of life, also increasing anxiety and depression. The prevalence of constipation in subjects with SCI is 20-58% (Ng et al., 2005). It is well known that constipation in SCI is due to prolonged colonic transit time. In SCI the extrinsic neural control is lost with an altered sympathic function (Winge et al., 2003). There is a clear association between constipation and the presence of a higher level of injury, as demonstrated by a mouth-to-cecum transit time prolonged in quadriplegics rather than paraplegics (Rajendran et al., 1992). Patients with cauda equina lesions may have an atonic bowel and develop severe and chronic constipation (Winge et al., 2003).

The variation in constipation prevalence in patients with different levels of neurologic deficit are related to different factors, such as attenuated gastrocolonic reflex, weakness of abdominal and perineal musculature, anorectal dysfunction and body immobilization (Stark et al., 1999; Ng et al., 2005).

Treating constipation in SCI subjects can be demanding. The usual management is a combination of bulking agents and scheduled enemas. Bowel training is used to evacuate the colon at regular intervals and an adequate fiber and fluid intake maintains bowel movements in a soft and bulky form. Shortly after breakfast, a rectal suppository and digital stimulation of the anorectum are used to induce reflex evacuation. These treatments usually leads to a daily planned evacuation. When they fail, prokinetic agents, parasympathetic nerve stimulators or colostomy can be used (Stark et al., 1999). In selected patients, transanal irrigation improves bowel function, compared with conservative management (Christensen et al., 2006).

5. Constipation in Parkinson Diseases (PD)

Bowel dysfunction is the most commonly observed non-motor feature of PD and it is a major factor in determining quality of life, progression of disability and nursing care (Hely et al., 2005). Some authors found constipation in 29% of patients (Edwards et al., 1991). However this symptom is under-recognised and under-treated but it has the potential to be more debilitating than motor features. The reason of this could be the patients' unawareness that these symptoms are linked to PD. Constipation is frequently reported as a prominent complaint before the onset of motor symptoms in about 50% of patients (Wood et al., 2010). Recently, an epidemiological study revealed an association between frequency of bowel movements and the risk of developing PD. Those patients with an initial finding of constipation were at a 3-fold increased risk of developing PD after 10 years from the initial report of constipation (Abbott et al., 2001). Bowel dysfunction can occur across all stages of PD but often occurs earlier during disease course and it might precede motor symptoms onset by more than a decade, correlating closely with the progression of Lewy pathology (Korczyn et al., 1990; Chaudhuri et al., 2009).

Bowel dysfunction can consist of both slowed colonic transit with consequent reduced bowel-movement frequency and difficulty with the act of defecation itself with excessive straining and incomplete emptying (anorectal dysfunction). Anorectal dysfunction is the more prevalent form of bowel impairment in PD Recognition can lead to earlier and potentially more effective therapeutic intervention (Pfeiffer et al., 2003).

An efficient and successful defecation requires the coordinated contraction and relaxation of several muscles. Defecography, anorectal manometry and analsphincter electromyography have been used to study defecation in PD, showing different abnormalities (Stocchi 2000). In a group of patients, anorectal dysfunction caused a paradoxical contraction of voluntary sphincters during defecation, which is believed to be a type of focal dystonia (Mathers et al., 1989).

Control of gastrointestinal function is complex and involves components of the central, autonomic, and enteric nervous systems (Pfeiffer et al., 2003). Changes in parasympathetic autonomic supply to the gut could certainly account for the impairment of gastrointestinal function in PD but abnormalities in the enteric nervous system within the gut itself have also been identified, including both Lewy-body formation and loss of dopaminergic neurons (Pfeiffer et al., 2003).

Lewy body pathology in the myenteric plexus, leading to colonic sympathetic denervation, has long been recognized in patients with PD. Such pathologic changes are associated with prolonged intestinal transit time and constipation, symptoms believed to occur in ~80% of patients with PD (Jost et al., 1997). Recently, Politis et al. have suggested a dopaminergic contribution to several non-motor symptoms of PD, including autonomic dysfunction and constipation (Politis et al., 2008).

Apomorphine treatment can improve anorectal dysfunction in PD and suggests that abnormalities of defaecation and anorectal function could be a consequence of dopamine deficiency secondary to the pathological changes of PD (Chaudhuri et al., 2009).

Medications used to treat the motor symptoms of PD (levodopa, anticholinergics) have even been implicated in further slowing of gastrointestinal motility and exacerbation of gastrointestinal dysfunction (Wood et al., 2010).

6. Assessment of constipation

A carefully taken history, including ongoing drugs and physical examination may be adequate in most cases. To perform more specific tests depend on single cases. It is possible to evaluate different aspects of bowel dysfunction. Measurement of whole gut transit time, swallowing a radio-opaque contrast medium, is the most widely used, non-invasive and inexpensive method to quantify large bowel function (Gill et al., 1994; Prokesch et al., 1999; Nicoletti et al., 1992; Evans et al., 1992). Anorectal function and pelvic floor incoordination can be assessed by anorectal testing, anorectal manometry and a balloon expulsion test. For instance, in this way it has been possible to demonstrate pelvic floor incoordination in MS patients (Diamant et al., 1999; et al., Weber 1987; Jameson et al., 1994; Chia et al., 1996). To evaluate distal colon innervation, electrical rectal sensory testing is a useful tool. It can distinguish between constipation connected to impaired central innervation of the gut or idiopathic form (Kamm et al., 1990).

7. Pharmacological therapies

Several drugs are available for patients with chronic constipation, ranging from older over-the-counter laxatives to more recently developed prescription drugs (Lembo 2003; Longstreth 2006; Ramkumar et al., 2005; Rao et al., 2009; Tack et al., 2009; Tramonte et al., 1997). Laxatives stimulate defecation by decreasing stool consistency and/or by stimulating colon motility. There are different classes of laxative drugs with different mechanism of action: osmotic laxatives and stimulant laxatives, bulking agents, stool softeners (Ramkumar et al., 2005; Tramonte et al., 1997).

8. Fibers

Fibers intake such as eating high-fiber foods (fruits, vegetables) or taking fiber/bulk supplements (bran, psyllium, methylcellulose or polycarbophil) is recommended during the initial treatment of constipation (Lembo et al., 2003; Locke et al., 2000). Unfortunately a long treatment (about 2-3 months) is required to obtain symptom relief. Despite the widespread use of fiber supplementation, this approach is effective in only a subset of patients and clinical trial supporting the use of increased fiber intake is limited.

9. Osmotic laxatives

Osmotic laxatives (poorly absorbed/non-absorbed sugars, saline laxatives and polyethylene glycol [PEG]) cause intestinal water secretion and may be recommended when fiber therapy is ineffective (Lembo et al., 2003). Many osmotic laxatives require few days to be effective and can result in electrolyte and volume overload in patients with renal or cardiac failure (Lembo et al., 2003). Osmotic laxatives can induce abdominal cramping, bloating and flatulence.

Osmotic agents are ions or molecules that are poorly absorbed by intestine and therefore they cause water retention in the intestinal lumen. Small intestine and colon are not able to keep an osmotic gradient between luminal contents and plasma, in contrast to stomach. Osmotic agents include: incompletely absorbed salts such as magnesium, sulphate and phosphate salts; sugar alcohols such as sorbitol or mannitol; poorly absorbed disaccharides such as lactulose and polyethylene glycol (PEG).

These agents keep water in intestinal lumen, increasing stool frequency, softening their consistency and decreasing straining. Non-absorbable sugars induce little improvement in stool frequency and consistency, but they cause colonic fermentation and consequently bloating and abdominal distention. Sodium sulphate reduces water absorption, stimulating peristalsis.

Bisodic phosphate is partially absorbed into the small bowel and it is well tolerated even if hyperphosphatemia can be observed as a consequence of overdose.

Magnesium hydroxide and magnesium salts improve stool frequency and consistency. Their systemic absorption is limited and the most common side effects are electrolyte abnormalities (i.e. hypokalemia and sodium overload) and diarrhea. In this light, magnesium should be used with great care in patients with hearth or/and renal failure and in the elderly (Golzarian et al., 1994; Schiller et al., 2001; Spinzi et al., 2007).

Lactulose is a complex sugar that is not digested and metabolized by bowel bacteria to form lactic, acetic and formic acids. In this way, it causes acidification of intestinal lumen, water secretion, production of H_2 and CO_2, and colon distension. Lactulose is very effective but induces flatulence and borborygmuses; moreover, its use should be avoided in patients with lactose intolerance.

In a systematic review of controlled trials, PEG was more effective than lactulose (Lee-Robichaud et al., 2010). PEG preparations are available with or without electrolyte supplements, and at different doses.

Macrogol 3350 is a mixture of non-absorbable polymers with high molecular weight. It is not metabolized by bowel bacteria and it works as a pure osmotic agent by keeping water into colon, causing rehydration and softer stool. The amount of water and electrolytes carried by macromolecular structure of macrogol is related to dose. The presence of electrolytes reduces risk of electrolyte imbalance, increasing safety in patients with kidney diseases (Migeon-Duballet et al., 2006). Moreover, macrogol causes less flatulence compared to lactulose, and it is useful for treating chronic constipation and drug-induced constipation (Di Palma et al., 2007; Zangaglia et al., 2007). Preparations containing electrolytes can also be used with high water volumes intake, such as for colon cleansing prior to colonoscopy or surgery (Di Palma et al., 2002; Szojda et al., 2007).

Glycerine is a well tolerated laxative, available just for rectal use. It works mainly by osmotic mechanism and stimulates evacuation lubricating stool.

Class	Active principle	Daily dose	Latency effect (hours)
Osmotic laxatives	Magnesium citrate	18g	0.5-3
	Magnesium hydroxide	2-4 g	6-8
	Magnesium sulfate	5-10g	6-8
	Sodium phosphate	10-20 ml / os 100ml/rectal	6-8 0.5-3
Sugars	Lactulose	5-30g	24-48
	Lactitol	10-15 g	24-48
	Sorbitol	5-15 g	24-48
	Mannitol	3-20 g	2-8
	PEG	15-40 g	24-48
	Glicerina	1-3 g	0.5
Diphenylmethane derivatives	Bysacodil	5-15 mg	10-12
	Sodium picosolfate	5-15 mg	6-10
Anthraquinone derivatives	Senna	24-48 mg	6-12
	Cascare	150-400 mg	6-12
	Rhubarb	50-100 mg	6-12
	Aloe	100-200 mg	6-12
	Frangola	200-600 mg	6-12
Surfactants	Docusate sodium	240 mg	0.5
Castor oil		15-60 ml	2-6

Table 1. Classification of laxative drugs

Stimulant laxatives (diphenylmethane and anthraquinone derivatives) produce rhythmic bowel contractions and should be recommended when osmotic laxatives fail (Borum et al., 2001). These agents increase intestinal motility and secretion after few hours from ingestion, but they may cause severe side effects (e.g. abdominal cramps, rebound constipation, damage to intestinal smooth muscles or enteric nervous system, colorectal cancer risk, hyponatremia, hypokalemia, dehydration. (Borum et al., 2001; Lembo et al., 2003; Muller-Lissner et al., 2005).

Several drugs and herbal preparations induce defecation by different mechanisms and are called 'stimulant' laxatives because they are able to stimulate bowel motility (Geboes et al., 1993). It is now clear that they have effect on mucosal transport as well as motility (Schiller et al., 1997).

These agents include: surface active agents, such as docusate and bile acids; diphenylmethane derivatives, such as phenolphthalein and bisacodyl; ricinoleic acid; anthraquinones, such as senna and cascara. Senna and bisacodyl cause rhythmic contractions of intestinal muscles, increasing bowel motility; moreover they increase water secretion into bowel. Bisacodyl is hydrolyzed in both small intestine and colon into a free-form that inhibits water absorption, but it also has an effect on enteric nervous system, inducing peristaltic response. Therefore, it should be avoided in patients with suspected intestinal obstruction. It is not clear whether these laxatives can induce damage to myenteric plexus, whereas it is known that their chronic use is associated with colonic melanosis that is reversible with drug withdrawal (about 5-6 months).

Bisacodyl and picosulfate are both phenylmethane prodrugs, hydrolysed by colonic bacteria or brush border enzymes to their active metabolite bis-(p-hydroxyphenyl)- pyridyl-2-methane (BHPM) which stimulates peristalsis.

The cathartic activity of bisacodyl and sodium picosulphate may depend on their conversion to compounds with free diphenolic groups (Sund et al., 1981).

Phenolphthalein inhibits water absorption in small intestine and colon by effecting prostaglandins, kinins and the $Na^{+}K^{+}$-ATPase pump. Phenolphthalein is absorbed and can be undergone to an enterohepatic circulation which may prolong its effect. It has been withdrawn from sale in the United States because some studies in rodents suggested it may be carcinogenic (Garner et al., 2000; Josefson et al., 1997). Adverse reactions of derivatives of diphenylmethane are cramping and abdominal pain; high doses induce severe diarrhea, electrolyte depletion, damage to enterocytes, skin allergies and Stevens-Johnson syndrome (phenolphthalein).

Docusates are ionic detergents which were designed to allow water to interact more effectively with stool solids, thereby softening stools. Bile acids are natural detergents that have been used as components of proprietary laxative preparations. If exogenous bile acid is taken orally, normal ileal absorptive capacity may be enormous and sufficient bile acid may get to the colon to reduce water and electrolyte absorption or to stimulate water secretion.

Anthraquinones are a group of chemicals based on tricyclic anthracene nucleus. They are produced by different plants. Monoanthrones can form dianthrones and can be conjugated with sugars to yield glycosides. They are pro-drugs, not absorbed in small intestine and hydrolyzed by colon bacteria to active forms. The effects on water secretion with increased fecal water may appear about 6-8 hours after administration. These compounds are indicated to treat chronic constipation. Adverse drug reactions include allergies, loss of body fluid and electrolytes, reversible melanosis.

The laxative action of Castor oil is due to an irritant action on tenuous intestine by rinoleic acid released by hydrolysis of triglycerides by pancreatic lipase. It has several action mechanisms:

- Na^{+}-K^{+}-ATPase inhibition
- cAMP levels increasing
- mucose permeability increasing
- NO synthesis

Castor oil is used to preparation bowel for diagnostic or surgical procedures. Adverse reactions include abdominal-cramps and intestinal wall damage (e.g. erosion of the mucosa and epithelial desquamation).

10. Stool softeners

Laxatives which mostly soften or lubricate stools (e.g. sodium dioctyl sulfosuccinate and liquid paraffin) seem to be more effective than placebo to increase bowel movement frequency. Liquid paraffin, since it may interfere with absorption of fat-soluble vitamins, should be avoided in patients with oropharyngeal dysphagia (Gondouin et al., 1996).

11. Bulk lassatives

Undigestible fibres attract water, causing larger and softer fecal mass, increasing bowel movements by 1.4 per week (Ramkumar et al., 2005; Tramonte et al., 1997). Fibres are usually well tolerated, although some symptoms, such as bloating, may get worse.

12. Neuromuscular agents

Some patients with colonic inertia seem to have a reduction in cholinergic nerve activity. This could be due to a damage to the enteric nervous system or to agents with anti-cholinergic effects. In such instances it would be useful to increase cholinergic stimulation of colonic smooth muscle by supplying a cholinergic agonist agent. Bethanechol can be used for this purpose with good results in some patients. Neostigmine has recently been suggested as effective therapy for acute colonic pseudo-obstruction.

13. 5-HT4 receptor agonists

Serotonin (5-HT) is a regulator of gastrointestinal motility, secretion and sensitivity. Through 5-HT4 receptors, mainly expressed in enteric neurons, 5-HT triggers and coordinates intestinal peristalsis (Gershon et al., 2007). Cisapride, a 5-HT4 receptor agonist, is used to stimulate gastrointestinal motility in patients with gastro-esophageal reflux disease, functional dyspepsia and gastroparesis; in 2000, it was withdrawn from sale because of the occurrence of fatal arrhythmia's through QT interval prolongation in patients with predisposing conditions (Tonini et al., 1999).

Tegaserod, a 5-HT4 receptor agonist is shown to be effective for treatment of irritable bowel syndrome with constipation (Al-Judaibi et al., 2010). In 2007, Tegaserod was withdrawn from the commerce because of increased risk of cardiovascular adverse events such as myocardial infarction, unstable angina and stroke (De Maeyer et al., 2008).

Prucalopride, a 5-HT4 receptor agonist, is a highly selective compound. It enhances colonic transit in healthy control subjects and in patients with chronic constipation, in a dose-dependent way (Bouras et al., 1999; Bouras et al., 2001; Camilleri et al., 2008; De Maeyer et al., 2008). It has been approved in Europe for the treatment of chronic constipation in women who do not respond to laxatives (2 mg). Recommended dose in elderly patients is 1 mg for a larger bio-availability (Müller-Lissner et al., 2010).

The misoprostol affects intestinal transit in healthy subjects and in patients with chronic constipation by stimulating water secretion and intestinal muscle contraction, especially in the left colon. Initial dosage should be 200 mcg twice/day, increased to 4/day, being sure it does not appear abdominal cramps.

14. Colonic secretagogues

Lubiprostone, the last drug approved by FDA for treatment of adult patients with chronic idiopathic constipation (Bethesda et al., 2006), is a gastrointestinal system-targeted bicyclic functional fatty acid that acts as a selective chloride channel (ClC-2) activator in the apical membrane of gastrointestinal epithelium to increase intestinal water secretion (Orr et al., 2006; Winpenney et al., 2005). This enhanced secretion of chloride leads to an increased intraluminal fluid amount, which facilitates transit in the intestine and thereby stool passage (Camilleri et al., 2006).

Lubiprostone, approved by FDA in 2006, is not yet approved in Europe (Drossman et al., 2009). Nausea, diarrhea and headache represent the most common adverse events, but patients also reported abdominal distension, abdominal pain and flatulence. Nausea can be reduced taking lubiprostone with food (Bethesda et al., 2006).

Linaclotide is a 14-amino acid peptide analog of guanylin and acts as an agonist at the luminal guanylin receptor on enterocytes, the guanylate cyclase-C receptor, which induces intestinal chloride and fluid secretion through cyclic GMP production (Bharucha et al., 2010). It is not yet approved for treatment of chronic constipation (Kurtz et al., 2006).

The mixed 5-HT4 receptor agonist/5-HT3 receptor antagonist renzapride relieves symptoms of constipation by softening stool consistency and increasing colonic transit. It has been tested only in patients with irritable bowel syndrome and constipation (Camilleri et al., 2004). Other 5-HT4 agonists, such as norcisapride and mosapride (Cremonini et al., 2005), neurotrophic factors (Coulie et al., 2000) and probiotic agents (Koebnick et al., 2003; Ouwehand et al., 2002) are also under investigations. Additional works are needed to determine their role in the treatment of chronic constipation.

Neurotrophins stimulate the development, growth and function of the nervous system, and increase colonic transit when administered subcutaneously in healthy subjects and patients with chronic constipation (Coulie et al., 2000).

Colchicine, usually used in the treatment of acute gout, induces diarrhea through an unknown dose-dependent mechanism. Colchicine increases stool frequency and reduces number of rescue laxatives needed. In a controlled trial, colchicine (1 mg/day) improved constipation in patients with slow transit (Taghavi et al., 2010).

15. Opiate antagonists

Opiate antagonists have also been suggested to treat constipation. These agents block opiate receptors in intestine avoiding mucosal absorption and inhibition of intestinal transit, caused by opiate. Thus mucosal absorption should be reduced and intestinal transit should be increase by the administration of drugs like naloxone and naltrexone. An early report suggested a role for this type of agent in idiopathic constipation, but a successive report denied it (Ragavan et al., 1983; Fotherby et al., 1987).

Opiate antagonists are useful in patients with opiate-induced constipation (Meissner et al., 2000; Yuan et al., 2000). The opiate antagonists methylnaltrexone and alvimopan are under investigation for the treatment of opiate-induced constipation and postoperative ileus, but unlike other opiate antagonists, they do not have any impact on central analgesia (Camilleri et al., 2005; Yuan et al., 2004). Their usefulness in treating non-opioid-induced constipation remains unclear.

16. Management of constipation in neurological disorders

Managing bowel function is a main concern in neurological patients, having an impact equal to mobility impairment on quality of life (Norton et al., 2010). It is important to get information on current bowel status in order to provide an effective treatment (Gulick et al., 2011). The frequent coexistence of faecal incontinence represents a challenge in the management of constipation (Hinds et al., 1990). On the other hand, treatment of constipation is essential, because constipation itself may worsen bladder symptoms (Hinds et al., 1989). Treatment of bowel dysfunction in MS patients is often empirical and there are a few studies comparing the efficacy of different measures such as high fibre diet, adequate intake of fluids, bowel habits, physical exercise and the use of medication (Winge et al., 2003).

Increasing dietary fibre may be useful in MS patients to soften faeces, but it is not helpful in patients with severe constipation, as observed in spinal cord injury (Cameron et al., 1996). Furthermore the need for adequate fluid intake when taking bulking agents should be strongly encouraged. Sufficient or additional fluid intake and the use of docusate stool softener (up to 600 mg/day) are simple ways to help maintain soft bowel movements (DasGupta et al., 2003). On the other hand, a high fibre diet or the use of bulking agents may produce increased symptoms connected to the presence of increased fermentable substrate if peristalsis is impaired (Winge et al., 2003; Muller et al., 1988).

Stimulant or osmotic laxatives are useful when transit is slow. Senna and bisacodyl are effective and their dose can be modulated in order to avoid faecal incontinence, an effect reported more frequently with osmotic laxatives (Gattuso et al., 1994; Schiller et al., 1999).

Rectal stimulants such as glycerine or bisacodyl suppository, sodium citrate micro-enema or phosphate enema, have the advantage of predictability in terms of time of response as observed in patients with spinal cord injury or stroke (House et al., 1997; Munchiando et al., 1993).

Pelvic floor incoordination has been observed in MS patients (Mathers et al., 1990; Weber et al., 1987; Chia et al., 1996). Behavioural therapies - the so called biofeedback - have an important role in the management of constipation in this group of patients and they are effective in subjects with mild to moderate disability and a non progressive disease course. Over a third of patients considered themselves to have benefited in the medium term, but long term effects of biofeedback are unknown. There are no physiological test that can predict the response to this treatment (Wiesel et al., 2000; Munteis et al., 2008). Biofeedback improves pelvic floor function, conditioning the voluntary striated muscle sphincter response and patient's consciousness of a stimulus distending the rectum (Wiesel et al., 2000; Storrie et al., 1997).

Recently, in a randomized controlled study, some authors have suggested a beneficial effect of abdominal massage on constipation symptoms in MS patients (McClurg et al., 2011). Abdominal massage decreases severity of constipation and abdominal pain, and increases bowel movements. In health subjects with constipation, the massage has a delayed effect that may occur first after a number of weeks so that it is considered a long-term treatment. It does not lead to decrease in laxative intake, so abdominal massage could be a complement to medication rather than a substitute (Lämås et al., 2009).

For selected patients with severe constipation, when there is a lack of response to conservative therapies, colostomy or the Malone appendicostomy can be contemplated (Wiesel et al., 2001; Hennessey et al., 1999; Krogh et al., 2009).

In stroke patients Early physical activity should be recommended for stroke patients to prevent new-onset constipation (Su et al., 2009). The establishment of dedicated stroke units with early mobilisation, rehydration and diet regulating measures have resulted in a remarkable reduction of the problems related to constipation in stroke patients (Winge et al., 2003; Cardin et al., 2010; Kumar et al., 2010). A systematic assessment of bowel habits by nursing staff with a simple practice-based approach towards bowel management and patient/caregiver education has been shown to be helpful in patients with stroke (Harari et al., 2004).

A step by step approach, from simple to more complex treatment measures, is strongly recommended also in PD patients. Increasing daily fibre and fluid intake is the first step, since it is deficient in many patients with PD. Fibre supplements with psyllium or methylcellulose is useful and it significantly increases stool frequency and weight. The second step is to add a stool softener, such as docusate. Then patient can use an osmotic laxative, such as lactulose or sorbitol. Also the regular use of polyethylene glycol electrolyte balanced solutions is effective. It would be better to avoid irritant laxatives and enemas, even if they could be useful in selected cases (Pfeiffer et al., 2003).

Intrajejunal infusion of duodopa in patients with advanced-stage PD determine an improvement in constipation and other bowel symptoms in addition to other non-motor symptoms (Chaudhuri et al., 2009). Treatment of defecatory dysfunction in PD is more demanding. Laxatives do not improve the impaired anorectal muscular coordination and may increase the problem. Dopaminergic drugs may be useful, being observed an improvement in anorectal manometric during "on" periods, with deterioration when "off"' (Pfeiffer et al., 2003). Also apomorphine therapy can improve anorectal dysfunction in PD (Chaudhuri et al., 2009). Botulinum-toxin injections into the puborectalis muscle have been used successfully in the treatment of parkinsonian defecatory dysfunction. Faecal incontinence is a potential complication. Behavioural treatment approaches such as biofeedback training have not been specifically investigated in PD (Pfeiffer et al., 2003).

17. Conclusions

Bowel dysfunction is a frequent complication in neurological disorders and it can be due to neurological lesions or non-neurological causes. Owing to a complex physiopathology and to the involvement of autonomic system, a specific treatment is limited. A multimodal approach is needed to manage symptoms successfully and to provide individualized care for a particular patient. It is essential to determine realistic aims. Training bowel habits associated with physical activity, proper use of medication and biofeedback, just for selected patients, is an effective strategy to improve constipation in neurologic patients for some time, depending largely on disability level. Bowel management is still often empirical in neurological disorders and well-designed controlled trials are needed.

18. References

[1] Abbott RD, Petrovich H, White LR, et al. Frequency of bowel movements and the future risk of Parkinson' s disease. *Neurology* 2001;57:456 - 62.

[2] Al-Judaibi B, Chande N, Gregor J. Safety and efficacy of tegaserod therapy in patients with irritable bowel syndrome or chronic constipation. *Can J Clin Pharmacol* 2010; 17(1):e177-93.
[3] American Gastroenterological Association. Guidelines on constipation. *Gastroenterology* 2000;119:1761-78.
[4] Bakke A, Myhr KM, Gronning M, et al. Bladder, bowel and sexual dysfunction in patients with multiple sclerosis–a cohort study. *Scand J Urol Nephrol Suppl* 1996;179:61–6.
[5] Bharucha AE, Waldman SA. Taking a lesson from microbial diarrheagenesis in the management of chronic constipation. *Gastroenterology* 2010;138(3):813–7.
[6] Borum ML. Constipation: evaluation and management. *Prim Care.* 2001; 28(3):577-90
[7] Bouras EP, 2001 Bouras EP, Camilleri M, Burton DD, Thomforde G, McKinzie S, Zinsmeister AR. Prucalopride accelerates gastrointestinal and colonic transit in patients with constipation without a rectal evacuation disorder. *Gastroenterology* 2001;120(2):354–60.
[8] Bouras EP, Camilleri M, Burton DD, McKinzie S. Selective stimulation of colonic transit by the benzofuran 5HT4 agonist, prucalopride, in healthy humans. *Gut* 1999;44(5):682–6.
[9] Bracci F, Badiali D, Pezzotti P, Scivoletto G, Fuoco U, Di Lucente L, Petrelli A, Corazziari E. Chronic constipation in hemiplegic patients. *World J Gastroenterol* 2007;13(29):3967-72.
[10] Cameron KJ, Nyulasi IB, Collier GR, Brown DJ. Assessment of the effect of increased dietary fibre intake on bowel function in patients with spinal cord injury. *Spinal Cord* 1996; 34:277-83.
[11] Camilleri M, Bharucha AE, Ueno R, Burton D, Thomforde GM, Baxter K, et al. Effect of a selective chloride channel activator, lubiprostone, on gastrointestinal transit, gastric sensory, and motor functions in healthy volunteers. *Am J Physiol Gastrointest Liver Physiol* 2006 May;290(5):G942–7.
[12] Camilleri M. Alvimopan, a selective peripherally acting mu-opioid antagonist. *Neurogastroenterol Motil* 2005;17:157–165.
[13] Camilleri M, Kerstens R, Rykx A, Vandeplassche L. A placebo-controlled trial of prucalopride for severe chronic constipation. *N Engl J Med* 2008;358:2344–54.
[14] Cardin F, Minicuci N, Teggia Droghi A, Inelmen EM, Sergi G, Terranova O. Constipation in the acutely hospitalized older patients. *Archives of Gerontology and Geriatrics* 2010;50:277-81.
[15] Chaudhuri KR, Schapira AHV. Non-motor symptoms of Parkinson's disease: dopaminergic pathophysiology and treatment. *Lancet Neurol* 2009; 8: 464–74.
[16] Chellingsworth M. Constipation as a presenting symptom of multiple sclerosis. *Lancet* 2003;362:1941.
[17] Chia YW, Gill KP, Jameson JS, Forti AD, Henry MM, Swash M, et al. Paradoxical puborectalis contraction is a feature of constipation in patients with multiple sclerosis. *J Neurol Neurosurg Psychiatry* 1996; 60:31-5.
[18] Christensen P, Bazzocchi G, Coggrave M, Abel R, Hultling C, Krogh K, Media S, Laurberg S. A randomized, controlled trial of transanal irrigation versus conservative bowel management in spinal cord–injured patients. *Gastroenterology* 2006;131:738–47.

[19] Coulie B, Szarka LA, Camilleri M, Burton DD, McKinzie S, Stambler N, et al. Recombinant human neurotrophic factors accelerate colonic transit and relieve constipation in humans. *Gastroenterology* 2000;119(1):41–50.
[20] Crayton H, Heyman RA, Rossman H. A multimodal approach to managing the symptoms of multiple sclerosis. *Neurology* 2004;63(Suppl 5):S12-S18.
[21] Cremonini F, Talley NJ. Treatments targeting putative mechanisms in irritable bowel syndrome. *Nat Clin Practice Gastroenterol Hepatol* 2005;2:82–88.
[22] DasGupta R, Fowler CJ. Bladder, bowel and sexual dysfunction in multiple sclerosis. Management strategies. *Drugs* 2003;63:153–66.
[23] De Maeyer JH, Lefebvre RA, Schuurkes JA. 5-HT4 receptor agonists: similar but not the same. *Neurogastroenterol Motil* 2008 Feb;20(2):99–112.
[24] De Seze J, Stojkovic T, Gauvrit JY et al. Autonomic dysfunction in multiple sclerosis: cervical spinal cord atrophy correlates. *J Neurol* 2001;248(4):297-303.
[25] Di Palma J, Smith J, Cleveland M. Overnight efficacy of polyethylene glycol laxative. *Am J Gastroenterol* 2002;97(7):1776–9.
[26] Di Palma JA, Cleveland MV, McGowan J, Herrera JL. A randomized, multicenter comparison of polyethylene glycol laxative and tegaserod in treatment of patients with chronic constipation. *Am J Gastroenterol* 2007;102(9):1964-71.
[27] Diamant NE, Kamm MA, Wald A, Whitehead WE. AGA technical review on anorectal testing techniques. *Gastroenterology* 1999; 116:735-60.
[28] Drossman DA, Chey WD, Johanson JF, Fass R, Scott C, Panas R, et al. Clinical trial: lubiprostone in patients with constipation- associated irritable bowel syndrome – results of two randomized, placebo-controlled studies. *Aliment Pharmacol Ther* 2009;29(3):329–41.
[29] Edwards LL, Pfeiffer RF, Quigley EMM, Hofman R, Baluff M. Gastrointestinal symptoms in Parkinson's disease. *Mov Disord* 1991; 6: 151–56.
[30] Evans RC, Kamm MA, Hinton JM, Lennard-Jones JE. The normal range and a simple diagram for recording whole gut transit time. *Int J Colorectal Dis* 1992; 7:15-17.
[31] Fotherby KJ, Hunter JO. Idiopathic slow-transit constipation: whole gut transit times, measured by a new simplified method, are not shortened by opioid antagonists. *Aliment Pharmacol Ther.* 1987;1(4):331-8.
[32] Fowler CJ. The cause and management of bladder, sexual and bowel symptoms in multiple sclerosis. *Baillieres Clin Neurol* 1997;6:447–66.
[33] Garner CE, Matthews HB, Burka LT. Phenolphthalein metabolite inhibits catechol-O-methyltransferase-mediated metabolism of catechol estrogens: a possible mechanism for carcinogenicity. *Toxicol Appl Pharmacol* 2000;162(2):124-31.
[34] Gattuso JM, Kamm MA. Adverse effects of drugs used in the management of constipation and diarrhoea. *Drug Safety* 1994; 10:47-65.
[35] Geboes K, Nijs G, Mengs U, Geboes KP, Van Damme A, de Witte P. Effects of 'contact laxatives' on intestinal and colonic epithelial cell proliferation. *Pharmacology* 1993;47(Suppl. 1):187–95.
[36] Gershon MD, Tack J. The serotonin signaling system: from basic understanding to drug development for functional GI disorders. *Gastroenterology* 2007;132(1):397–414.
[37] Gill KP, Chia YW, Henry MM., Shorvon PJ. Defecography in multiple sclerosis patients with severe constipation. *Radiology* 1994;191:553–6.

[38] Golzarian J, Scott Jr H, Richards W. Hypermagnesemia-induced paralytic ileus. *Dig Dis Sci* 1994;39(5):1138–42.
[39] Gondouin A, Manzoni P, Ranfaing E, Brun J, Cadranel J, Sadoun D, et al. Exogenous lipid pneumonia: a retrospective multicentre study of 44 cases in France. *Eur Respir J* 1996;9(7):1463–9.
[40] Guinet A, Jousse M, Damphousse M, Hubeaux K, Le Breton F, Ismael SS, Amarenco G. Modulation of the rectoanal inhibitory reflex (RAIR): qualitative and quantitative evaluation in multiple sclerosis. *Int J Colorectal Dis* 2011;26:507-513.
[41] Gulick EE. Bowel management related quality of life in people with multiple sclerosis: Psycometric evaluation of the QoL-BM measure. *Int J Nurs Stud* 2011; doi:10.1016/j.ijnurstu.2011.02.002.
[42] Haldeman S, Glick M, Bhatia NN, Bradley WE, Johnson B. Colonometry, cystometry and evoked potentials in multiple sclerosis. *Arch Neurol* 1982;39:698-701.
[43] Harari D, Norton C, Lockwood L and Swift C. Treatment of constipation and fecal incontinence in stroke patients: randomized controlled trail. *Stroke* 2004; 35:2549-55.
[44] Hely MA, Morris JG, Reid WG, Trafficante R. Sydney Multicenter Study of Parkinson's disease: Non-L-doparesponsive problems dominate at 15 years. *Mov Disord* 2005;20:190 - 99.
[45] Hennessey A, Robertson NP, Swingler R, Compston DAS. Urinary, faecal and sexual dysfunction in patients with multiple sclerosis. *J Neurol* 1999;246:1027-32.
[46] Hinds JP, Eidelman BH, Wald A. Prevalence of bowel dysfunction in multiple sclerosis. A population survey. *Gastroenterology* 1990;98, 1538–42.
[47] Hinds JP, Wald A. Colonic and anorectal dysfunction associated with multiple sclerosis. *Am J Gastroenterol* 1989;84:587–95.
[48] Hong KS, Kang DW, Koo JS, Yu KH, Han MK, Cho YJ, Park JM, Bae HJ, Lee BC. Impact of neurological and medical complications on 3-month outcomes in acute ischaemic stroke. *European Journal of Neurology* 2008,15:1324-31.
[49] House JG, Stiens SA. Pharmacologically initiated defecation for persons with spinal cord injury: effectiveness of three agents. *Arch Phys Med Rehabil* 1997; 78:1062-65.
[50] Jameson JS, Rogers J, Chia YW, Misiewicz JJ, Henry MM, Swash M. Pelvic floor function in multiple sclerosis. *Gut* 1994; 35:388-90.
[51] Josefson D. US to ban sale of many laxatives over the counter. *BMJ* 1997 ;315(7109):627.
[52] Jost WH. Gastrointestinal motility problems in patients with Parkinson' s disease. Effects of antiparkinsonian treatment and guidelines for management. *Drugs Aging* 1997;10:249 - 58.
[53] Kamm MA, Lennard-Jones JE. Rectal mucosal electrosensory testing - evidence for a rectal sensory neuropathy in idiopathic constipation. *Dis Colon Rectum* 1990; 33:419-23.
[54] Koebnick C, Wagner I, Leitzmann P, Stern U, Zunft HJ. Probiotic beverage containing Lactobacillus casei Shirota improves gastrointestinal symptoms in patients with chronic constipation. *Can J Gastroenterol* 2003;17:655–659.
[55] Korczyn AD. Autonomic nervous system disturbances in Parkinson' s disease. *Adv Neurol* 1990;53:463 - 68.
[56] Krogh K, Christensen P. Neurogenic colorectal and pelvic floor dysfunction. *Best Pract Res Clin Gastroenterol* 2009;23(4):531-43.
[57] Kumar S, Selim MH, Caplan LR. Medical complications after stroke. *Lancet Neurol* 2010;9:105-18.

[58] Kurtz C, Fitch D, Busby RW, Fretzen A, Geis GS, Currie MG. Effects of multidose administration of MD-1100 on safety, tolerability, exposure, and pharmacodynamics in healthy subjects [abstract] *Gastroenterology* 2006;130:A-26.

[59] Lacy BE, Levy LC. Lubiprostone: a chloride channel activator. *J Clin Gastroenterol* 2007 Apr;41(4):345–51.

[60] Lämås K, Lindholm L, Stenlund H, Engström B, Jacobsson C. Effects of abdominal massage in management of constipation - A randomized controlled trial. *International Journal of Nursing Studies* 2009;46:759-67.

[61] Lawthom C, Durdey P, Hughes T. Constipation as a presenting symptom. *Lancet* 2003;362:958.

[62] Lee-Robichaud H, Thomas K, Morgan J, Nelson RL. Lactulose versus polyethylene glycol for chronic constipation. *Cochrane Database Syst Rev* 2010 Jul 7 (7):CD007570.

[63] Lembo A, Camilleri M. Chronic constipation. *NEJM* 2003;349:1360–8.

[64] Longstreth GF, Thompson WG, Chey WD, et al. Functional bowel disorders. *Gastroenterology* 2006;130:1480–91.

[65] Mark ES. Challenging problems presenting as constipation. *Am J Gastroenterol* 1999;94:567-74.

[66] Mathers SE, Ingram DA, Swash M. Electrophysiology of motor pathways for sphincter control in multiple sclerosis. *J Neurol Neurosurg Psychiatry* 1990;53:955-60.

[67] Mathers SE, Kempster PA, Law PJ, et al. Anal sphincter dysfunction in Parkinson's disease. *Arch Neurol.* 1989; 46:1061–64.

[68] McClurg D, Hagen S, Hawkins S, Lowe-Strong A. Abdominal massage for the alleviation of constipation symptoms in people with multiple sclerosis: a randomized controlled feasibility study. *Mult Scler* 2011;17(2):223-33.

[69] Meissner W, Schmidt U, Hartmann M, Kath R, Reinhart K. Oral naloxone reverses opioid-associated constipation. *Pain* 2000;84(1):105-9.

[70] Migeon-Duballet I, Chabin M, Gautier A, Mistouflet T, Bonnet M, Aubert JM, et al. Long-term efficacy and cost-effectiveness of polyethylene glycol 3350 plus electrolytes in chronic constipation: a retrospective study in a disabled population. *Curr MedRes Opin* 2006;22(6):1227–35.

[71] Müller-Lissner S, Rykx A, Kerstens R, Vandeplassche L. A double-blind, placebo-controlled study of prucalopride in elderly patients with chronic constipation. *Neurogastroenterol Motil* 2010 Sep;22(9):991–8.

[72] Muller-Lissner SA. Effect of wheat bran on weight of stool and gastrointestinal transit time: a meta analysis. *Br Med J Clin Res Ed* 1988; 296:615-17.

[73] Munchiando JF, Kendall K. Comparison of the effectiveness of two bowel programs for CVA patients. *Rehabil Nurs* 1993; 18:168-72.

[74] Munteis E, Andreu M, Martinez-Rodriguez J, Ois A, Bory F, Roquer J. Manometric correlations of anorectal dysfunction and biofeedback outcome in patients with multiple sclerosis. *Mult Scler* 2008;14(2):237-42.

[75] Ng C, Prott G, Rutkowski S, Li Y, Hansen R, Kellow J, Malcolm A. Gastrointestinal symptoms in spinal cord injury: relationships with level of injury and psychologic factors. *Dis Colon Rectum* 2005;48:1562–68.

[76] Nicoletti R, Mina A, Balzaretti G, Tessera G, Ghezzi A. Intestinal transit studied with radiopaque markers in patients with multiple sclerosis. *Radiol Medica* 1992; 83:428-30.

[77] Nordenbo AM, Andersen JR, Andersen JT. Disturbances of ano-rectal function in multiple sclerosis. *J Neurol* 1996;243:445–51.

[78] Norton C, Chelvanayagam S. Bowel problems and coping strategies in people with multiple sclerosis. *Br J Nurs* 2010;19(4):220, 221-6.
[79] Orr KK. Lubiprostone: a novel chloride channel activator for the treatment of constipation. *Formulary*. 2006;41:118–120.
[80] Ouwehand AC, Lagstrom H, Suomalainen T, Salminen S. Effect of probiotics on constipation, fecal azoreductase activity and fecal mucin content in the elderly. *Ann Nutr Metab* 2002;46:159–162.
[81] Pfeiffer RF. Gastrointestinal dysfunction in Parkinson's disease. *Lancet Neurol* 2003;2:107-16.
[82] Politis M, Piccini P, Pavese N, Brooks DJ. Evidence of dopamine dysfunction in the hypothalamus of patients with Parkinson's disease: an in vivo 11C-raclopride study. *Exp Neurol* 2008; 214: 112–16.
[83] Prokesch RW, Breitenseher MJ, Kettenbach J, et al. Assessment of chronic constipation: colon transit time versus defecography. *Eur J Radiol* 1999;32:197–203.
[84] Ragavan VV, Wardlaw SL, Kreek MJ, Frantz AG. Effect of chronic naltrexone and methadone administration on brain immunoreactive beta-endorphin in the rat. *Neuroendocrinology* 1983;37(4):266-8.
[85] Rajendran SK, Reiser JR, Bauman W, Zhang RL, Gordon SK, Korsten MA. Gastrointestinal transit after spinal cord injury: effect of cisapride. *Am J Gastroenterol* 1992;87:1614-7.
[86] Ramkumar D, Rao SS. Efficacy and safety of traditional medical therapies for chronic constipation: systematic review. *Am J Gastroenterol* 2005;100(4):936–71.
[87] Rao SSC. Constipation: evaluation and treatment of colonic and anorectal motility disorders. *Gastrointest Endosc Clin N Am Clinics North America* 2009;19:117–39.
[88] Robain G, Chennevelle JM, Petit F, Piera JB. Incidence of constipation after recent vascular hemiplegia: prospective cohort of 152 patients. *Rev Neurol (Paris)* 2002;158:589-92.
[89] Sakakibara R, Yamaguchi C, Uchiyama T, Ito T, Liu Z, Yamamoto T, Awa Y, Yamanishi T, Hattori T. Pelvic autonomic dysfunction without paraplegia: a sequel of spinal cord stroke. *Eur Neurol* 2008;60:97-100.
[90] Saunders DR, Sillery J, Rachmilewitz D, Rubin CE, Tytgat GN. Effect of bisacodyl on the structure and function of rodent and human intestine. *Gastroenterology* 1977;72(5 Pt 1):849-56.
[91] Schiller LR, Santa Ana CA, Porter J, Fordtran JS. Validation of polyethylene glycol 3350 as a poorly absorbable marker for intestinal perfusion studies. *Dig Dis Sci* 1997 Jan;42(1):1-5.
[92] Schiller LR. Clinical pharmacology and use of laxatives and lavage solutions. *J Clin Gastroenterol* 1999; 28:11-18.
[93] Schiller LR. Review article: the therapy of constipation. *Aliment Pharmacol Ther* 2001;15(6):749-63.
[94] Spinzi GC. Bowel care in the elderly. *Dig Dis* 2007;25(2):160-5.
[95] Stark ME. Challenging Problems Presenting as Constipation. *Am J Gastroenterol* 1999;94:567–74.
[96] Stocchi F, Badiali D, Vacca L, et al. Anorectal function in multiple system atrophy and Parkinson's disease. *Mov Disord* 2000; 15: 71–6.
[97] Storrie JB. Biofeedback: a first-line treatment for idiopathic constipation. *Br J Nurs* 1997; 6:152-8.

[98] Su Y, Zhang X, Zeng J, Pei Z, Cheung RTF, Zhou Q, Ling L, Yu J, Tan J, Zhang Z. New-Onset Constipation at Acute Stage After First Stroke: Incidence, Risk Factors, and Impact on the Stroke Outcome. *Stroke* 2009;40:1304-9.

[99] Sund RD, Olsen G. Net sodium and glucose transport in the jejunum, ileum and colon of anaesthetized rats in response to intraluminal theophylline and anionic surfactants. *Acta Pharmacol Toxicol (Copenh)* 1981 Jul;49(1):65-71.

[100] Swash M. Sphincter disorders and the nervous system. In: Aminoff MJ (3rd ed). Neurology and general medicine. Churchill Livingstone 2001: 537-55.

[101] Szojda MM, Mulder CJ, Felt-Bersma RJ. Differences in taste between two polyethylene glycol preparations. *J Gastrointestin Liver Dis* 2007;16(4):379–81.

[102] Tack J, Müller-Lissner S. Treatment of chronic constipation: current pharmacologic approaches and future directions. *Clin Gastroenterol Hepatol* 2009 May;7(5):502–8.

[103] Taghavi SA, Shabani S, Mehramiri A, Eshraghian A, Kazemi SM, Moeini M, et al. Colchicine is effective for short-term treatment of slow transit constipation: a double-blind placebo-controlled clinical trial. *Int J Colorectal Dis* 2010;25(3): 389–94.

[104] Taylor MC, Bradley WE, Bhatia N, Glick M, Haldeman S. The conus demyelination syndrome in multiple sclerosis. *Acta Neurol Scand* 1984; 69:80-9.

[105] Tonini M. Polyethylene glycol as a non-absorbable prokinetic agent in the lower gastrointestinal tract. *Ital J Gastroenterol Hepatol* 1999;31 Suppl 3:S238-41.

[106] Tramonte S, Brand M, Mulrow C, Amato M, O'Keefe M, Ramirez G. The treatment of chronic constipation in adults: a systematic review. *J Gen Intern Med* 1997;12(1):15–24.

[107] Ullman T, Reding M. Gastrointestinal dysfunction in stroke. *Semin Neurol* 1996;16:269-75.

[108] Weber J, Grise P, Roquebert M, Hellot MF, Mihout B, Samson M, et al. Radiopaque markers transit and anorectal manometry in 16 patients with multiple sclerosis and urinary bladder dysfunction. *Dis Colon Rectum* 1987; 30:95-100.

[109] Wiesel PH, Norton C, Glickman S, Kamm MA. Pathophysiology and management of bowel dysfunction in multiple sclerosis. *Eur J Gastroenterol Hepatol* 2001;13:441-8.

[110] Wiesel PH, Norton C, Roy AJ, Storrie JB, Bowers J, Kamm MA. Gut focused behavioural treatment (biofeedback) for constipation and faecal incontinence in multiple sclerosis. *J Neurol Neurosurg Psychiatry* 2000;69:240-3.

[111] Winge K, Rasmussen D, Werdelin LM. Constipation in neurological diseases. *J Neurol Neurosurg Psychiatry* 2003;74:13–19.

[112] Winpenny JP. Lubiprostone. *IDrugs* 2005;8(5):416-22.

[113] Wolters EC. Non-motor extranigral signs and symptoms in Parkinson's disease. *Parkinsonism Relat Disord* 2009 Dec;15 Suppl 3:S6-S12.

[114] Wood LD, Neumiller JJ, Setter SM, Dobbins EK. Clinical review of treatment options for select non-motor symptoms of Parkinson's disease. *Am J Geriatr Pharmacother* 2010;8:294-315.

[115] Yuan CS, Foss JF. Antagonism of gastrointestinal opioid effects. *Reg Anesth Pain Med* 2000;25(6):639-42.

[116] Yuan CS, Wei G, Foss JF, O'Connor M, Karrison T, Osinski J. Effects of subcutaneous methylnaltrexone on morphine-induced peripherally mediated side effects: a double-blind randomized placebo-controlled trial. *J Pharmacol Exp Ther* 2002;300:118–123

[117] Zangaglia R, Martignoni E, Glorioso M, Ossola M, Riboldazzi G, Calandrella D, Brunetti G, Pacchetti C. Macrogol for the treatment of constipation in Parkinson's disease. A randomized placebo-controlled study. *Mov Disord* 2007;22(9):1239-44.

9

Bowel Dysfunction in Persons with Multiple Sclerosis

Elsie E. Gulick[1] and Marie Namey[2]
[1]*Rutgers, The State University of New Jersey,*
[2]*Mellen Center for MS Treatment & Research Cleveland Clinic,*
USA

1. Introduction

Information is presented pertaining to the characteristics of multiple sclerosis (MS) including bowel dysfunction that consists of constipation, fecal incontinence or both constipation and fecal incontinence. Bowel functions and its neural control, prevalence and symptoms of constipation and fecal incontinence that is characteristic of persons with MS together with a description of procedures for assessment and intervention strategies are presented. The outcomes of bowel interventions and their effects on the quality of life of persons with MS together with suggestions for further research are also presented.

2. Characteristics of Multiple Sclerosis

Multiple Sclerosis (MS) is an inflammatory and demyelinating autoimmune disorder (Herndon, 2003) that affects approximately 2.5 million people worldwide (Moses, Picone & Smith, 2008) that has an approximately 2:1 female to male ratio (Willer, Dyment, Risch, Sadovnick, & Ebers, 2003). This disease of the central nervous system (CNS) affects nerve pathways in the brain and spinal cord. MS is thought to be acquired through the complex interaction of genetic and environmental factors (Goodin, 2010). Environmental influences are thought to include low levels of ultraviolet radiation and vitamin D, viruses, and non infectious agents such as smoking and psychological stress (Milo & Kahana, 2010; Sloka, Silva, Pryse-Phillips, Meta & Wee Yong, 2011; Carlye, 1997; Mehta, 2010; Koch-Henrikson & Sorensen, 2010).

The onset of MS generally occurs during young adulthood (Weinshenker, 1993) and is usually characterized by an initial relapsing and remitting course followed by a progressive course (Wienshenker, 1998; Vukusic & Confavreux, 2007). As a result of impairment of the CNS bowel dysfunction is one of many symptoms experienced by persons with MS that consists of constipation and fecal incontinence. Constipation, defined as two or fewer bowel movements per week, the need to manipulate the rectum digitally to facilitate defecation all or most of the time, and/or use of laxatives, enemas, or suppositories more than once a week, has a prevalence rate between 43% and 73% in the MS population (Hinds, Eidelman & Wald, 1990; Nordenbo, Andersen, & Andersen, 1996). Fecal incontinence, defined as uncontrolled or involuntary emissions of flatus and/or stools, has a prevalence of between 51% and 53% in the MS population (Hinds et al. 1990; Nordenbo et al. 1996).

3. Bowel functions and neural control

Principal functions of the colon include 1) absorption of water and electrolytes from the chime, ingested food that is mixed with stomach secretions that pass into the small intestine and on to the large intestine, and 2) storage of fecal matter until it can be expelled (Guyton & Hall, 2006). Mixing movements known as haustrations promote absorption of fluid and dissolved substances causing the chime to become a semisolid slush. Haustral contractions propel the material in the colon toward the rectum. Beginning of the transverse colon and continuing to the sigmoid, mass movements mainly take over the propulsive role which occur only one to three times each day and most frequently for 15 minutes during the first hour after eating breakfast. Mass movements are facilitated by the gastrocolic and duodenocolic reflexes that result from distention of the stomach and duodenum via extrinsic nerves of the autonomic nervous system. When a mass movement forces feces into the rectum, the desire for defecation is normally initiated, including reflex contraction of the rectum and relaxation of the anal sphincters. Loss of fecal matter through the anus is prevented by tonic contraction of the internal and external anal sphincters. The external sphincter is controlled by nerve fibers in the pudendal nerve which is under voluntary conscious control. Defecation is initiated by defecation reflexes and is fortified by the parasympathetic defecation reflex that involves the sacral segments of the spinal cord. Conscious relaxation of the internal sphincter and forward movement of feces toward the anus normally initiate contraction of the external sphincter which prevents defecation and if kept contracted defecation reflexes die out after a few minutes and remain quiescent for several hours or until additional amounts of feces enter the rectum (Guyton & Hall, 2006).

The autonomic nervous system, consisting of sympathetic and parasympathetic nerve fibers, controls the visceral functions pertaining to gastrointestinal mobility and secretion and is activated mainly by centers located in the spinal cord, brain stem and hypothalamus (Guyton & Hall, 2006). Sympathetic nerves originate in the spinal cord between segments T-1 and L-2 and pass from here into the sympathetic chain and then to the tissue and organs that are stimulated by the sympathetic nerves. Sympathetic fibers from cord segments T-7 through T-11 pass into the abdomen. Sympathetic nerve endings secrete norepinephrine and have two major types of adrenergic receptors: alpha and beta. Alpha receptors cause intestinal relaxation, intestinal sphincter contraction, and bladder sphincter contraction. Beta receptors cause intestinal and uterus relaxation and bladder wall relaxation. Autonomic reflexes that inhibit gastrointestinal activity that severely block movement of food through the intestines are initiated by sensory signals that pass to the prevertebral sympathetic ganglia or to the spinal cord and then are transmitted through the sympathetic nervous system back to the gut (Guyton & Hall, 2006).

Parasympathetic fibers leave the CNS through cranial nerves III, VII, IX, and X; and the second and third sacral spinal nerves; and the first and fourth sacral nerves (Guyton & Hall, 2006). The vagus, cranial nerve X, supplies parasympathetic nerves to the proximal half of the colon. The sacral parasympathetic fibers congregate in the pelvic nerves which leave the sacral plexus at S-2 and S-3 levels and distribute their peripheral fibers to the descending colon, rectum, and external genitalia. Parasympathetic nerve endings secrete acetylcholine which increases the overall activity of the gastrointestinal tract by promoting peristalsis and relaxing the sphincters to allow rapid propulsion of contents along the tract and is associated with increases in rates of secretion by many of the gastrointestinal glands.

However, strong sympathetic stimulation inhibits peristalsis and increases the tone of the sphincters resulting in greatly slowed propulsion of food through the tract and sometimes decreases secretion as well (Guyton & Hall, 2006). Figure 1 illustrates bowel anatomy and neural components associated with bowel function.

Hypothalamic centers can control gastrointestinal activity. Thus, autonomic centers in the brain stem act as relay stations for control of activities initiated at higher levels of the brain. Higher areas of the brain can alter all or portions of the autonomic system to cause constipation.

4. Constipation

Constipation can be primary or secondary (Candelli, Nista, Zocco, & Gasbarrini, 2001). Primary constipation, also known as idiopathic or functional constipation, is considered when no definite cause is found and specific diseases cannot be demonstrated. Constipation is considered secondary when specific causes are recognized such as poor fiber diet, intestinal neoplasm, drugs, or specific diseases such as multiple sclerosis. Constipation in MS patients can be caused either by slow colonic transit, abnormal rectal function, or abnormal pelvic floor function (Chia, Fowler, Kamm, Henry, Lemieux & Swash, 1995; DasGupta & Fowler, 2003; Weber, Grise, Roquebert, Hellot, Mihout, Samson, Beuret-Blanquart, Pasquis &Denis, 1987).

Slow transit constipation is characterized by prolonged delay in the transit of stool through the colon due to a primary dysfunction of the colonic smooth muscle or its nerve innervations (Rao, 2007). Symptoms may include straining during defecations, lumpy or hard stools, sensation of incomplete evacuation of stool, sensation of anorectal obstruction of stool, and manual maneuvers to facilitate defecation. Pathologic conditions include phasic colonic motor activity; diminished gastrocolonic response following a meal; the high amplitude, prolonged duration, propagated contractions are decreased; and the velocity of propagation is slower, waves have a greater tendency to abort prematurely, and their amplitude is also decreased (Rao, 2007). Weber et al. (1987) in a study of 16 MS patients reported that transit times of radiopaque markers led to an objective confirmation of constipation in 13 of the 15 patients. Interruption of sympathetic innervations from the dorsolumbar spinal cord via the superior mesenteric ganglion and vagal parasympathetic innervations to the right colon together with sympathetic innervations from the dorsolumbar spinal cord via the inferior mesenteric ganglion and parasympathetic innervations from the sacral spinal cord via the erigentes nerves to the left colon were proposed to explain the decreased transit observed in MS patients (Weber et al. 1987). Wald (1986) reported that prolonged transit time throughout the entire colon among MS patients responded poorly to treatment compared to those characterized by slow transit restricted to the left colon or delay only through the anorectal structures.

Abnormal rectal function, also known as dyssynergic defecation, obstructive defecation, anismus, pelvic floor dyssynergia, or outlet obstruction, is characterized by difficulty to expel stool from the anorectum (Rao, 2007). Symptoms include the need to strain excessively, feeling of incomplete evacuation, abdominal fullness or bloating, and need to use fingers to facilitate defecation (Rao, Tuteja, Vellema, Kempf & Stessman, 2004). Dyssynergic defecation may be caused by paradoxical anal contraction or involuntary anal spasm during defecation

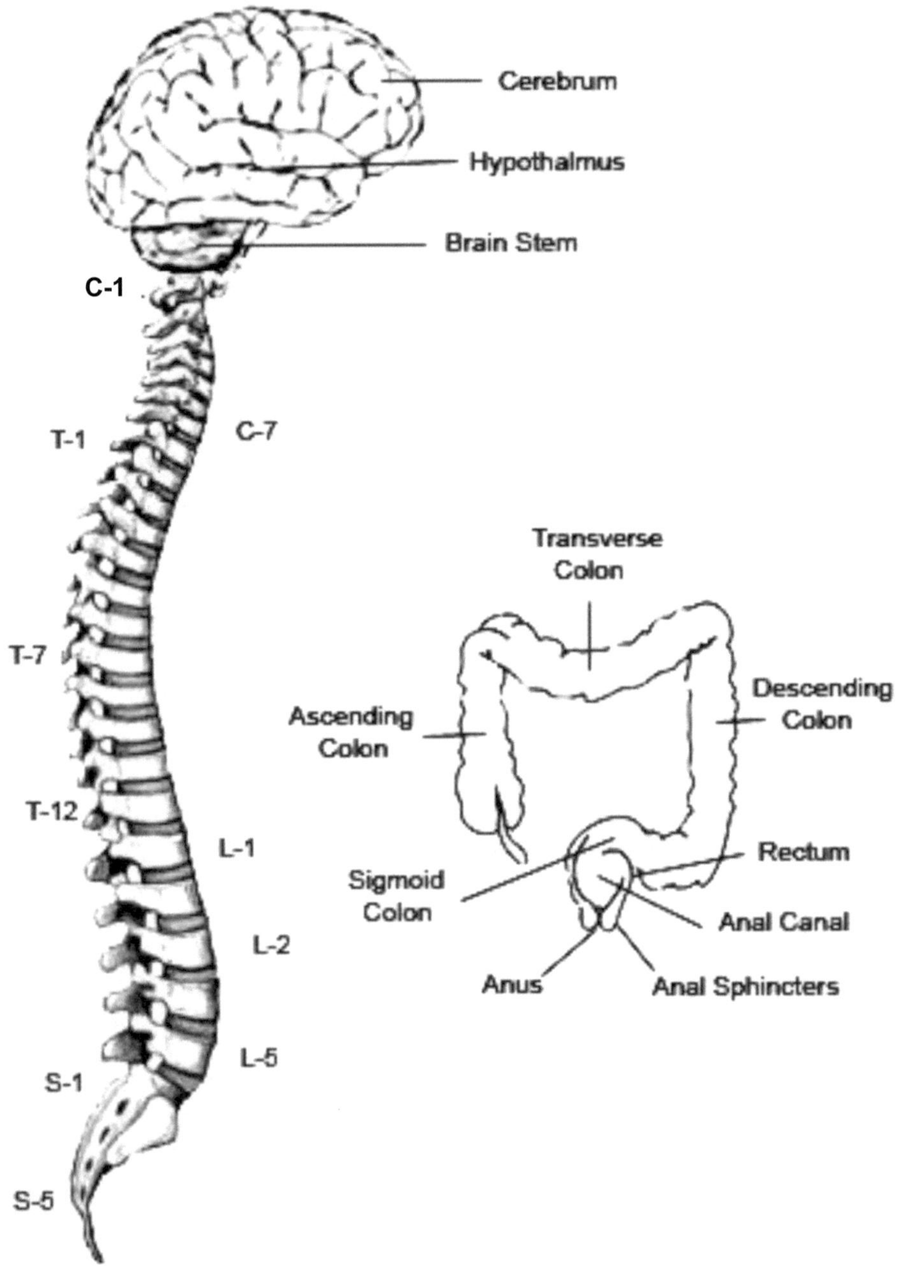

Fig. 1. Bowel anatomy and neural components associated with bowel function

(Rao, 2007). Munteis, Andreu, Martinez-Rodriquez, Ois, Bory & Roquer, (2008) reported that 32 MS patients with constipation compared to 22 patients without neurological or gastroenterologic abnormalities had significantly lower squeeze maximal sphincter pressure and higher anal inhibitory reflex, conditions that impede defecation. Women with pelvic organ prolapse and who reported chronic straining to defecate reportedly have a high risk for constipation (Arya, Novi, Shaunik, Morgan & Bradley, 2005). The authors theorized that chronic straining may produce weakness of the pelvic floor resulting in pudendal nerve injury with loss of tonicity of pelvic floor muscles and subsequent development of prolapse.

5. Fecal incontinence

Fecal incontinence is characterized by an urgent need to defecate and loss of stool. Major factors causing fecal incontinence among MS patients include the lack of voluntary control of the external anal sphincter, rectal hyperreactivity, reduced rectal tone and contractility causing fecal impaction and rectal distension, and reduced or lost anal sensibility (Chia, et al. 1995; Hennessey, Robertson, Swingler & Compston, 1999; Krogh & Christensen, 2009). Studies among persons with MS have shown that fecal incontinence is associated with reduced rectal sensation, a markedly reduced external sphincter function, weakness of pelvic floor musculature and an inability to close the anorectal angle (Nordenbo, et al. 1995; Waldron et al. 1993). Causes of fecal incontinence unrelated to MS include diarrheal infections due to viral, bacterial, and protozoal agents (Walker, 2006); food allergy (Walker, 2006); or pudendal nerve damage associated with childbirth (Swash, Snooks & Chalmers, 1987).

6. Assessment of bowel dysfunction

Bowel problems particularly fecal incontinence is often withheld from sharing the problem with health care providers due to feelings of embarrassment or shame (Khan, Pallant, Shea & Whishaw, 2009; Powell & Rigby, 2000; Wald, 2007). Therefore, since bowel dysfunction is relatively common among persons with MS it is important for health care providers to ask their MS patients in a careful supportive manner about their bowel function as accurate assessment of the presenting bowel problem is key to the successful treatment and management of bowel dysfunction (Irwin, 2003). Important bowel assessment information needed by the health care provider can be obtained through periodically patient-administered surveys and/or through patient interviews. A description of several patient-administered survey questionnaires are described below.

6.1 Instruments used to assess bowel function/dysfunction

Patient-administered questionnaires regarding their bowel function or dysfunction can provide health care providers with information that can assist them in determining appropriate treatment, counseling, or needed referrals. Periodic assessments are important to determine if the current treatment is effective or in need of change. Periodic assessments are also needed because of possible change in the patient's disability status that may increase bowel problems (Wiesel, Norton, Glickman, & Kamm, 2001). Several patient-administered questionnaires are described below.

6.1.1 The Bowel Function Questionnaire for Persons with Multiple Sclerosis (BFQ-MS)

The BFQ-MS, developed for persons with MS, is a patient-administered scale that consists of 15 items pertaining to constipation, 13 items pertaining to fecal incontinence and 20 items pertaining to both constipation and fecal incontinence (Gulick, 2010). The questionnaire items inquire about one's medical/surgical background that may be related to bowel dysfunction; medications with constipating or diarrheal effects; symptoms (frequency, consistency, time spent on the toilet, amount of time once the urge is felt before defecation occurs, skin breakdown around anus or perineum, pain/discomfort on defecation, flatulence, strain to defecate, feel bowel is not empty after defecation); nondrug interventions; drug interventions; and improvement or worsening over time. The items are rated on a Likert scale that ranges between 0 and 5 with higher scores indicating a worsening of bowel problems. Cronbach alpha reliability coefficients for the Constipation, Fecal Incontinence, and both Constipation and Fecal Incontinence subscales were 0.70, 0.68, and 0.69, respectively. The three subscales demonstrate satisfactory validity as they were able to differentiate symptom and treatment differences between the three types of bowel dysfunction.

6.1.2 The Quality of Life Scoring Tool Relating to Bowel Management (QOL-BM)

The QOL-BM, originally developed for use with spinal cord injured patients (Slater, 2003), was tested for reliability and validity with a sample of 502 persons with MS (Gulick, 2011). Principal component analysis and Varimax rotation factor analysis of the 11-item scale used with MS patients resulted in two factors: Management and Relationships. The 6-item Management subscale consists of items related to severity of bowel difficulty, convenience/inconvenience of bowel care, and satisfaction with bowel care. The 5-item Relationships subscale consists of items related to worry about bowel accidents, personal relationships and social activity. Internal consistency reliability for the total scale was 0.90 and was 0.86 for the Management subscale and 0.83 for the Relationships subscale suggesting satisfactory reliability. Discriminant validity was shown for the total and subscales based on the MS patient's disability level ($p < .05$).

6.1.3 Constipation Symptom Assessment Instrument (PAC-SYM)

The PAC-SYM is a constipation symptom assessment scale consisting of 12 items that measure stool symptoms, rectal symptoms and abdominal symptoms (Frank, Kleinman, Farup, Taylor & Miner, 1999). Items are rated on a 5-point Likert scale from absence of symptoms (0) to very severe (4). Internal consistency (Cronbach's alpha = 0.89) and test-retest reliability (intraclass correlation = 0.75) were high. Within subject change over a 6-week period demonstrated significantly improved scores. The PAC-SYM scale has been used with opium-induced constipation patients (Slappendel, Simpson, Dubois & Keininger, 2006) and with women with pelvic organ prolapse and constipation (Arya et al. 2005).

6.1.4 The Brief Fecal Incontinence Score

The Brief Fecal Incontinence Score is a 7-item scale that measures frequency of stool, stool consistency, flatulence, altered lifestyle, drug and nondrug interventions, and inability to defer defecation for 15 minutes (Vaizey, Carapeti, Cahill & Kamm, 1999). A five-point Likert rating scale from Never (0) to Daily (5) is used. The scale correlated closely with clinical assessment ($r=0.79$), showed high test-retest reliability ($r=0.87$), and showed sensitivity to change from pre-surgery to 6-weeks post-surgery ($p<0.004$) suggesting good reliability and validity. The scale has not reportedly been used with MS patients.

6.2 Patient interview regarding bowel function/dysfunction

One or more of the survey questionnaires could be used prior to conducting an interview with the patient. Suggested questions to be asked during the patient interview are described in Table 1. General questions are presented and depending on the individual's response more detailed questions can be explored.

A follow-up to the interview questions includes a physical assessment, described below, to determine if abnormalities of the anorectum and perineum can be detected.

6.3 Physical assessment and laboratory tests pertaining to bowel dysfunction

The following examinations are recommended to assist in identifying underlying causes of bowel dysfunction (Hinds & Wald, 1989; Irwin, 2002; Namey & Halper, 2000).

1. Abdominal assessment by palpating along the course of the colon to detect any mass or tenderness
2. Rectal and pelvic exam to look for prolapse, rectocele, hemorrhoids, fissures, and fecal impaction
3. Digital assessment of resting anal tone and external sphincter pressures
4. Digital assessment to obtain stool sample for testing for occult blood
5. Puborectalis function by hooking the examining finger posteriorly onto the puborectalis bar and feeling the muscle contract when the patient squeezes and relaxes when asked to strain
6. Check perineum for skin condition
7. Blood work should include blood glucose, electrolytes, calcium, and if necessary, thyroid function (Hinds & Wald, 1989)

Information obtained from the interview, physical assessment and blood work should guide the development of an individualized bowel program.

7. Interventions to control bowel function/dysfunction

7.1 Basic bowel program: Constipation

Development of the bowel program should be comprehensive and individualized to include the physical abilities of the patient, availability of care, the chosen lifestyle and preferences of the patient and education of the patient and caregiver (Coggrave, Wiesel & Norton, 2006). The approach to treating bowel problems in MS should be guided by an evaluation of likely pathophysiology of the bowel symptoms (Hay-Smith, Siegert, Weatherall & Abernethy, 2007). Simple and conservative approaches of a bowel program include appropriate diet and fluid intake, awareness of medications that may have a constipating or diarrheal effect, active or passive exercise, and toileting regime.

7.1.1 Diet and fluid intake

Good nutrition is vital for one's overall health and for a 1800 calorie diet the recommendations include a daily intake of 1 ½ cups of fruit, 2 ½ cups of dark green/orange/red vegetables, 6 ounces of grains, 5 ½ ounces of meat and beans, 3 cups of milk, 24 grams of oils, and 20-30 grams of fiber (Dietary Guidelines for Americans-2010). A

1. Tell me about your bowel movements during the past week.	
2. How frequently do you move your bowels during the week? Is this your typical pattern? Are you satisfied with this pattern?	
3. Are your bowel movements usually liquid, loose, soft, hard, lumpy or does the stool consistency vary?	
4. Now ask questions shown below according to reported stool consistency.	
Stools usually Liquid or Loose	**Stools Usually Hard or Lumpy**
1. Do you lose some or all of the stool before making it to the toilet? If yes, when and where does this occur?	1. Do you strain to pass your stool? If yes, what is the frequency?
2. What things have you done to help control loss of stool. Tell me about them.	2. Do you feel your bowel is not empty or need to go again quickly? If yes, what is the frequency?
3. Do you use medications to help you control loss of stool or bowel leakage? Tell me about them.	3. What things have you done to help you move your bowels? Tell me about them.
4. Do you have any food allergies? If yes, tell me about them.	4. Do you use laxatives, suppositories, or enemas to help with bowel care? Tell me about them.
Additional background questions to ask pertaining to possible causes of bowel dysfunction and toileting facilities	
1. How long have you experienced your bowel problem?	
2. What medications are you currently taking other than laxatives or anti-diarrheal agents?	
3. Tell me about the foods you usually eat and the type and amount of beverage each day.	
4. Do you experience pain or discomfort when moving your bowels?	
5. Do you need assistance from other persons to help you with bowel care?	
6. Are toilet facilities readily available and comfortable?	
7. How much does your bowel problem bother you and interfere with every day activities?	
8. Are there conditions that may be related to your current bowel problem?	
Surgical procedures: abdomen, rectal, anal, or perineum	
Difficult childbirth (woman)	
Medical conditions such as colitis, Crohns disease	
Failure to heed the urge to move your bowels	
Sexual abuse	
Medications with constipating or diarrheal effects	
9. Is there a family history of bowel problems?	
10. Is there anything else you'd like to tell me about your bowel problem?	

Table 1. Interview Regarding Bowel Functions/Dysfunctions

common cause of constipation is a diet low in fiber. Fiber may be soluble that dissolves easily in water and takes on a gel-like texture in the intestine or insoluble fiber that passes through the intestine almost unchanged. Together, the bulk and soft texture of fiber helps prevent hard, dry stools (Rigby & Powel, 2005). However, based on a meta-analysis of studies of the effect of fiber treatment on bowel function, Muller-Lissner (1988) concluded that there is no justification for claiming rye bran, a form of insoluble fiber, given to patients with constipation can return stool output and transit time to normal since there may be a motility disorder of the colon which is primary or secondary to an underlying disease or an altered lifestyle that is responsible for constipation.

The addition of high fiber foods to one's diet has mixed results. A study of 41 women with pelvic floor disorder given slow increases of high-fiber cereal until 28 grams were reached over a 42 day period resulted in withdrawal of 11 patients largely due to inability to tolerate the fiber diet (Shariati, Maceda & Hale, 2008). The 30 patients who completed the study reported significant decreases in adominal pain and bloating, painful bowel movements, rectal bleeding, incomplete bowel movements, consistency of stool, straining or squeezing, laxative use, vaginal and/or perineal splinting. Increasing fiber to one's diet should be introduced slowly in order to control for symptoms of bloating and gas. The addition of yoghurt containing Lactobacillus GG along with a fiber rich diet can decrease gastrointestinal symptoms associated with a fiber rich diet (Hongisto, Paajanen, Saxelin & Korpela, 2006). A list of fiber foods together with the standard serving size and grams of fiber identified by the USDA and USDHHS (2010) are presented in Table 2.

7.1.2 Medications that can adversely affect bowel dysfunction

Control of various MS-related symptoms or other non-MS conditions such as hypertension may require medications that have constipating affects. A list of these medications is shown in Table 3. Patients need to be queried about the medications that they currently are taking to determine if any of them have constipating and/or diarrheal effects.

7.1.3 Physical activity to promote bowel function

Body movement through exercise helps promote peristalisis of the colon, that may reduce the likelihood of constipation (Petajan , Gappmaier, White, Spencer, Mino & Hicks, (1996). Exercise may be passive or active depending on the disability status of the person with MS. Physical activity may be increased according to functional level by performing activities of daily living, pursuing more active recreation and eventually developing a structured exercise program (Petajan & White, 1999). Several studies with persons with MS given aerobic training and fitness (Petajan et al. 1996) or extended outpatient rehabilitation program (Di Fabio, Soderberg, Choi, Hansen & Schapiro,1998) demonstrated improvement in the study participants' bowel functioning. A study by Gulick and Goodman (2006) evaluated the effect of everyday activities performed in and around the home among 123 persons with MS ranging between mild to severe disability. After controlling for disability level, bowel and bladder symptoms increased with increased levels of physical activity.

7.1.4 Toileting regime to assist in bowel evacuation

A number of activities related to toileting can aid defecation. Planning the toileting routine during the first hour following breakfast takes advantage of increased peristalsis of the colon which moves the chime/feces into the sigmoid colon and rectum (Guyton & Hall, 2006). Patients who are able to sit safely and tolerate sitting on a commode or toilet for short

Food	Standard Portion Size	Dietary Fiber in Standard Portion (g)
Grains		
Bran ready-to-eat cereal (100%)	1/3 cup (about 1 ounce)	5.6-8.1
Plain rye wafer crackers	2 wafers	5.0
Bran ready-to-eat cereals (various)	1/3-3/4 cup (about 1 ounce)	2.6-5
Whole wheat English muffin	1 muffin	4.4
Soybeans, green, cooked	½ cup	3.8
Shredded wheat ready-to-eat cereal	½ cup (about 1 ounce)	2.7-3.8
Whole wheat spaghetti, cooked	½ cup	3.1
Oat bran muffin	1 small	3.0
Pearled barley, cooked	½ cup	3.0
Vegetables		
Artichoke, cooked	¼ cup hearts	7.2
Green peas, cooked	1/2 cup	3.5-4.4
Mixed vegetables, cooked	½ cup	4.0
Sweet potato, baked in skin	1 medium	3.8
Greens (spinach, collards, turnip greens), cooked	½ cup	2.5-3.5
Sauerkraut, canned	½ cup	3.4
Potato, baked, with skin	1 small	3.0
Broccoli, cooked	½ cup	2.6-2.8
Fruit		
Asian pear	1 small	4.4
Raspberries	½ cup	4.0
Blackberries	½ cup	3.8
Prunes, stewed	½ cup	3.8
Figs, dried	¼ cup	3.7
Apple, with skin	1 small	3.6
Banana	1 medium	3.1
Orange	1 medium	3.1
Strawberries	1 cup	3.0
Guava	1 fruit	3.0
Dates	¼ cup	2.9
Lentils and Nuts		
Beans (navy, pinto, black, kidney, white, great northern, lima), cooked	½ cup	6.2-9.6
Split peas, lentils, chickpeas, or cowpeas, cooked	½ cup	5.6-8.1
Soybeans, mature, cooked	½ cup	5.2
Almonds	1 ounce	3.5

Table 2. Selected Food Sources Ranked by Standard Food Portion and Amounts of Dietary Fiber

Drugs with Constipating Effects
Analgesics (including non-steriodal anti-inflammatory drugs)
Antacids (e.g., aluminum and calcium compounds)
Anticolinergics (e.g., Oxybutynin, Ditropan(R))
Anticonvulsants (e.g., oxcarbazepine, Trileptal(R))
Antidepressants (e.g., selective serotonin reuptake inhibitors)
Antihypertensives (e.g., clonidine, Catapres(R))
Antimotility (e.g., Loperamide, Imodium(R))
Anti-Parkinsonism (e.g., Sinemet, Carbidopa, Lodosyn(R))
Antispastic (eg.Clonide, Catapres(R))
Diuretics (e.g., hydrochlorothiazide)
Hematinics (e.g., Iron)
Laxatives (long term use)
Opiates (e.g., Morphine, Codeine)
Psychotherapeutic drugs (e.g., Thioridazine, Mellaril(R))
Drugs with Diarrheal Effects
Antacids containing magnesium
Antibiotics
Antidepressant (e.g., Sertraline, Zoloft(R))
Antihypertension (e.g., Captopril, Capoten(R))
Chemotherapy drugs
Nonsteroidal anti-inflammatory drugs, Ibuprofen, Motrin®

Table 3. Medications Containing Constipating or Diarrheal Effects

periods and lean forward to bring pressure onto the colon may promote defecation (Lewicky-Gaupp et al. 2008; Pierce et al. 2001). Toilet facilities must be readily accessible and comfortable. The need for toilet assistance from caretakers as well as their attitude towards bowel care needs to be assessed (Irwin, 2003).

7.2 Other components of a bowel program: Constipation

Some persons with MS may benefit from other forms of bowel control depending on their disability level and comfort of the particular procedure. These include abdominal massage, biofeedback, anal stimulation, digital removal of feces, and rectal or trans-anal irrigation. Various laxatives may be used and/or enemas. Gastroenterology referrals may be indicated for some persons with MS.

7.2.1 Abdominal massage

Abdominal massage reportedly aids peristalsis of the colon to enhance the mass movement of the gut and increases the strength of the contractions and propulsion force through sensory stimulation of the parasympathetic division (McClurg, Hagen, Hawkins & Lowe-Strong, 2010). This stimulation increases the mobility of the muscles to the gut, increases digestive secretions and relaxes the sphincters in the rectoano region. McClurg, using abdominal massage instruction over a four week period given to 15 MS patients compared to 15 MS patient controls with an EDSS disability score between 2.5-6.0 (mean = 3.5) resulted in improved frequency of defecation from 2 to 4.5 defecations per week, decreased time spent defecating from 10 minutes to 6 minutes for the experimental group compared to 12 to 10 minutes per day for the control group. Consistency of stools for both the experimental and control groups was softer at the end of the four week period compared to baseline.

7.2.2 Biofeedback for constipation

Biofeedback represents a number of behavioral modification techniques, which, when applied to treatment of constipation and fecal incontinence, may include sphincter exercises, bowel habit retraining, counseling, health education and use of medications (Wiesel, Norton, Roy, Storrie, Bowers & Kamm, 2000). In a study of 18 persons with MS given biofeedback instruction for anorectal dysfunction, improvement was shown in 8 (44.4%) of the MS patients given biofeedback who had milder manometric abnormalities (squeeze maximal sphincter pressure, anal inhibitory reflex, and paradoxical contraction of the puborectal musculature) and limited disability (Munteis et al. 2008).

7.2.3 Anal stimulation

The defecation reflex can be stimulated by dilating the anus with a lubricated gloved finger. This procedure stimulates the anal sigmoid reflex which causes the colon to contract, the anus relaxes, and fecal contents can be pushed out and is most effective if performed when the patient is in a sitting position (Pierce, et al. 2001).

7.2.4 Digital removal of feces

Digital removal of feces may be performed by patients themselves or by nurses who have received specialized training in the performance of digital removal of feces (Kyle, et al. 2005). However, this procedure should only be used as the last resort and after all other methods of bowel evacuation have failed (Powell & Rigby, 2000). Because of the invasive nature of the procedure patient consent is needed for health care providers to perform the procedure.

7.2.5 Rectal or trans-anal irrigation

This procedure involves a process of facilitating evacuation of feces from the bowel by passing water or other liquids in to the bowel via the anus in a quantity sufficient to reach beyond the rectum (Coggrave, 2008). The infused water distends the rectal wall and stimulates the stretch receptors to stimulate defecation (Pellatt, 2007).

7.2.6 Laxatives, suppositories and enemas

Persons with MS use a range of interventions to help manage the symptoms of constipation, fecal incontinence and/or both constipation and fecal incontinence, with varying degrees of success. A list of medications used for constipation together with their action and either precautions or contraindications (Curry Jr. & Butler, 2006) are presented in Table 4. Close monitoring of the frequency and duration of laxative use can be beneficial in determining whether normal bowel habits are reestablished between bouts of constipation or if a more severe condition exists (Curry & Butler, 2006).

7.2.7 Gastroenterology referrals

Although most patients with chronic constipation can usually be treated successfully in the primary care setting, some patients may require referral to a gastroenterologist. Reasons for referral include suspicion of defecatory disorders such as pelvic floor dyssynergia, lack of sufficient response to empiric treatment, and worsening of symptoms despite treatment (Bleser, 2006). Objective testing for bowel dysfunction include Anorectal Manometry, the Balloon Expulsion Test, Defecography and Colonic Transit Studies.

Anorectal Manometry is used to assess basal pressure in the rectum and anal canal, squeeze maximal sphincter pressure, rectal sensation, simulated defecation, inhibitory reflex, and presence of paradoxical contraction of the puborectal musculature (Munteis et al. 2008). The Balloon Expulsion Test is used to quantify the ability of a patient to evacuate a water-filled (usually 50 ml) balloon. It can serve as a functional marker in biofeedback programs for pelvic floor retraining (Gill, Chia, Henry & Shorvon, 1994; Locke III, Pemberton & Phillips, 2000). Defecography includes the scintigraphic method used to evaluate anorectal angulation and pelvic floor descent during evacuation. Barium defecography is performed in conjunction with a standard enema. These tests can determine failure of the anorectal angle to open and degree of pelvic floor descent during defecation (Locke, Pemberton & Phillips, 2000). Colonic Transit Studies are used to determine the rate at which fecal residue moves through the colon using radiopaque markers (Locke, Pemberton & Phillips, 2000). The test provides quantitative information about colonic transit, enables the identification and characterization of transit abnormality, and allows assessment of the severity of the problem (Ringel, 2003).

Medication	Action	Precautions or Contraindications
Bulk-forming Methylcellulose, Citrucel® Carboxymethyl cellulose sodium Malt soup extract, Maltsupex® Partially hyrdrolyxe guar gum Benerfiber® Polycarbophi, FiberCort®	Contain natural and semisynthetic hydrophilic polysaccharides and cellulose derivative that dissolve in the intestinal fluid to facilitate passage of the intestinal contents and stimulate peristalsis. Doesn't affect absorption of nutrients.	Abdominal cramping and flatulence may occur. Avoid taking a bulking agent within 1 to 2 hours of taking other medications. Drink at least 8 oz of fluid with each dose. Acts within 12 to 24 hours
Emollients/ Stool Softeners Docusate sodium, Colace® Docusate calcium Docusate potassium	Increase the wetting efficiency of intestinal fluid, promotes a softer stool, helps prevent painful defecation and straining.	May cause diarrhea and mild abdominal cramping. Avoid use if nausea, vomiting, or abdominal pain exist. Acts within 24 to 72 hr.
Lubricants Mineral Oil	Soften fecal contents by coating them, thus preventing colonic absorption of fecal water.	Excessive use may impair absorption of vitamins A, D, E, and K. Acts in 6 to 8 hours.

Medication	Action	Precautions or Contraindications
Saline Laxatives (Osmotics) Magnesium citrate, Citroma® Magnesium hydroxide, Milk of Magnesium® Magnesium sulfate, Epson Salts® Polyethylene Glycol, MiraLAX® Lactulose	Produce both secretory and motor reactions that draw water into the intestine, to increase intraluminal pressure which in turn increases intestinal motility.	Indicated for acute evacuation of the bowel. Take on an empty stomach as food will delay its action. May cause abdominal cramping, diuresis, nausea, vomiting, and dehydration. Acts within 30 minutes to 3 hours.
Stimulants Senna, Senokot® Bisacodyl Castor oil	Increase the propulsive peristaltic activity of the intestine by local irritation of the mucosa or by a more selective action on the intramural nerve plexus of intestinal smooth muscle, thus increasing motility. Stimulate secretion of water and electrolytes in either the small or large intestine or both.	Used for simple constipation, but not to be used for more than 1 week unless ordered by a physician. May cause severe cramping, electrolyte and fluid deficiencies, enteric loss of protein, malabsorption resulting from excessive hypermotility and catharsis, and hypokalemia. Usually acts within 6 to 12 hours or may require up to 24 hours.
Suppositories Glycerin Dulcolax	A hyperosmotic laxative that irritates the lining of the intestine. Draws water into the rectum to stimulate a bowel movement. Has a direct stimulating effect on the network of nerves in the large intestine. Provides lubrication to promote elimination of stool.	Do not use if abdominal pain, feel sick, or have vomiting. Take plenty of fluids while taking the medication. Usually acts within 30 minutes
Enemas Mineral Oil Fleet Enema	Lubricates the colon and allows for added cleansing. Pulls water from the body into the bowel which helps to soften the stool and cause a bowel movement.	Enema solutions can cause fluid and electrolyte disturbances in the blood if used on a chronic basis. May cause anal irritation, diarrhea, gas, nausea, stomach, cramps. Acts within 5 to 15 minutes.

Table 4. Medications used to Manage Constipation

7.3 Components of a bowel program: Fecal incontinence

As was noted for the Bowel Program described for constipation, the development of the bowel program for fecal incontinence should be comprehensive and individualized to include the physical abilities of the patient, availability of care, the chosen lifestyle and preferences of the patient and education of the patient and caregiver (Coggrave, et al. 2006). Except for fecal incontinence caused by viral, bacterial or protozoal infections, treatment for fecal incontinence commonly experienced by MS patients should entail a conservative approach. These include dietary considerations, medications that have diarrheal effects, toileting routine, incontinent pads, biofeedback, antidiarrheal medications and possibly anal plugs or sacral nerve stimulation.

7.3.1 Dietary considerations

Persons with MS could benefit from monitoring their food intake through use of a food diary to determine if certain foods may be related to fecal incontinence. A food diary should list what and how much one eats and when one has an incontinent episode to determine if a pattern between certain foods and incontinence occur. Known foods that have been associated with fecal incontinence include milk, egg, peanut, tree nuts, fish, shellfish, soy seeds, wheat, fruits and vegetables (Sicherer, 2011). Avoidance of fatty foods, foods rich in simple sugars, spicy foods, and caffeine may be helpful in controlling fecal incontinence (Walker, 2006). Hinds and Wald (1989) suggest reducing fiber intake if incontinence of solid stool occurs.

7.3.2 Medications associated with fecal incontinence

Medications given to control various MS-related symptoms and/or conditions unrelated to MS may contain diarrheal properties. Table 3 lists several of these medications.

7.3.3 Toileting regime to control fecal incontinence

Although patients are strongly encouraged to establish a daily time for defecation (DasGupta & Fowler, 2003) fewer than five percent of MS patients with fecal incontinence reported using a daily time for defecation (Gulick, 2010). Hinds and Wald (1989) suggest establishing a routine schedule of enemas or suppositories (e.g., once a week) to keep the rectum empty.

7.3.4 Use of incontinent pads

Incontinence pads have been shown to be used by approximately one third of MS patients who experience fecal incontinence (Gulick, 2010). Use of these pads can conceal the incontinence problem from others particularly if the quantity of lost stool is small. When soiling of the pad occurs, it needs to be changed in order to prevent skin breakdown of the perineum and/or buttocks that can result in incontinence dermatitis and/or pressure ulcers (Whitely, 2007).

7.3.5 Biofeedback for fecal incontinence

This intervention may be helpful by improving the strength of pelvic floor muscles and rectal sensory perception to improve anorectal coordination (Nordenbo, et al. 1996).

Biofeedback retraining is more successful in persons with MS with limited disability and a non-progressive disease course (Wiesel, et al. 2000).

7.3.6 Antidiarrheal medications

These medications remain the main treatment for fecal incontinence. In taking antidiarrheal medications patients need to be cautioned about the potential adverse effects of dehydration. Antidiarrheal medications have been shown to be used by approximately one third of MS patients who experience fecal incontinence (Gulick, 2010). Commonly used antidiarrheal medications (Walker, 2006) are shown in Table 5.

Medication	Action	Precautions and/or Contraindications
Loperamide, Imodium®	Slows intestinal motility, allowing absorption of electrolytes and water through the intestine and decreased gastro-intestinal secretion.	Occasional dizziness and constipation may occur. Infrequent occurrence of abdominal pain, abdominal distention, nausea, vomiting, dry mouth, fatigue, and hypersensitivity reactions.
Bismuth Subsalicylate, Kaopectate®	Reduces the frequency of unformed stools, increases stool consistency, relieves symptoms of abdominal cramping, and decreases nausea and vomiting.	Mild tinnitus is a dose-related side effect that may be associated with moderate to severe salicylate toxicity. Discontinue drug if tinnitus occurs. The drug may interact with other medications, such as aspirin, tetracycline and quinolone antibiotics.
Diphenoxylate/ Atropine, Lomotil®	Slows intestinal contractions and peristalisis allowing the body to consolidate intestinal contents and prolong transit time, thus allowing the intestines to draw moisture out of the intestinal material to stop the formation of loose or liquid stools.	Discontinue drug if one experiences extreme thirst, decreased urination, muscle cramps, or weakness.
Racecadotril Acetorphan Hidrasec®	Acts as a peripherally acting enkephalinase inhibitor that has an antisecretory effect by reducing secretion of water and electrolytes into the intestine	Shown to promptly and significantly reduce total stool output in 48 to 72 hours after initiation of treatment. Is well tolerated in adults and children.

Table 5. Medications used to Manage Fecal Incontinence

7.3.7 Anal plug

The anal plug has been developed to prevent loss of stool and is a disposable device for patients with anorectal incontinence. In a study of 10 patients with incontinence to gas and both liquid and solid stool the use of variable anal plugs for three consecutive weeks resulted in one patient withdrawing from the study due to discomfort of the anal plug, and for the remaining subjects there were no episodes of incontinence during 82% of time in which anal plugs were used with a median time of 7 to 12 hours depending on type of plug (Mortensen & Humphreys, 1991). Norton and Kamm (1999) evaluated two sizes of anal plugs each of which was tested for a two week period in a sample of 20 ambulatory and self-caring patients with intractable fecal incontinence for solid or liquid stool. Results indicated that the majority 14 (70%) could not tolerate a plug due to discomfort but for those that could tolerate the plug, it was highly successful at controlling fecal incontinence. Patients with neurogenic bowel dysfunction and have attenuated anorectal sensation may tolerate the presence of the anal plug (Emmanuel, 2010). Research is needed to determine if the use of anal plugs are helpful in controlling fecal incontinence in persons with MS.

7.3.8 Sacral Nerve Stimulation

Sacral nerve stimulation (SNS) for patients with severe fecal incontinence undergo implantation with a quadripolar electrode and pulse generator placed subcutaneously in the gluteal area (Tjandra, Chan, Yeh & Murray-Green, 2008). Compared to a control group who received medical therapy that comprised bulking agents, pelvic floor exercises, and dietary management, fecal incontinence was greatly improved with chronic SNS immediately after implantation and was sustained during the 12 month follow-up period in a randomized study of non-MS patients with severe fecal incontinence (Tjandra et al. 2008). Adverse events with SNS included pain at implant site which resolved after percutaneous aspiration and excessive tingling in the vaginal region. Research is needed to determine if the use of SNS is helpful in controlling fecal incontinence in persons with MS.

8. Outcome of various management strategies for bowel dysfunction in persons with MS

Possibly due to the multiplicity of causes of bowel dysfunction in persons with MS the outcome from the various treatment/intervention approaches have not yielded very satisfactory results. In a study of bowel dysfunction among persons with MS, Gulick (2010) noted that 54.1% (99/183) reported their constipation had worsened over time; 38.6% (22/57) reported their fecal incontinence worsened over time; and 71.8% (117/163) who experienced both constipation and fecal incontinence reported their constipation problem had worsened over time. Additionally, a survey of MS respondents who reportedly used a wide range of strategies to manage their bowel problems indicated that few of them were rated as very helpful (Norton & Chelvanayagam, 2010).

Many conditions and treatments that accompany MS over its long term illness trajectory may as a single entity or in combination lead to bowel dysfunction. These conditions frequently include ambulation difficulty, spasticity, fatigue, depression, urinary incontinence and various medications. In addition to MS related causes of bowel dysfunction there may be other health problems unrelated to MS that can cause bowel dysfunction.

Studies clearly acknowledge the adverse impact that bowel dysfunction has on the quality of life of persons with MS as the various bowel problems greatly interfere with the person's physical and social activities, family relationships, which also lead to the development of considerable emotional distress (Gulick, 1997; Norton & Chelvanayagam, 2010; Nortvedt, Riise, Frugard, Mohn, Bakke, Skar, Nyland, Glad & Myhr, 2007; Wollin, Bennie, Leech, Windsor, & Spencer, 2005). With regard to bowel dysfunction, persons with MS report that fecal incontinence has a significantly greater negative impact on their quality of life than constipation (Gulick, 2011; Norton & Chelvanayagam, 2010). Of the various MS related symptoms, respondents in the study by Norton and Chelyanayagam reported that bowel dysfunction and bowel management had the greatest negative impact on their quality of life.

9. Conclusion

Bowel dysfunction consisting of constipation and/or fecal incontinence is common in persons with MS. Causes of bowel dysfunction may be due to neurological lesions in the CNS or by non-neurological causes. The relapsing-remitting or progressive MS course may result in acute or chronic symptoms of constipation and/or fecal incontinence. Subjective and objective assessments of bowel symptoms using a team of specialists to determine the causes, appropriate treatment/intervention with ongoing monitoring of the condition is essential. Further studies with persons with MS are needed to determine the effectiveness of treatments/interventions given to improve bowel functions among those with bowel problems while controlling for confounding issues. Further study is also needed to determine the effectiveness of using objective laboratory procedures to identify or rule out specific causes of bowel problems.

10. References

Arya, L.A., Novi, J.M., Shaunik, A., Morgan, M.A. & Bradley C.S. (2005). Pelvic organ prolapse, constipation, and dietary fiber intake in women: A case-control study. *Americn Journal of Obstetrics and Gynecology,* Vol.192, pp.1687-1691.

Bleser, S.D. (2006). Chronic constipation: Let symptom type and severity direct treatment. *The Journal of Family Practice,* Vol.55, No.7, (July 2006), pp. 587-593.

Candelli, M., Nista, E.C., Zocco, M.A. & Gasbarrini, A. (2001). Idiopathic chronic constipation: Pathophysiology, diagnosis and treatment. *Hapato-Gastroenterology,* Vol.48, pp.1050-1057.

Carlye, I. P. (1997). Multiple sclerosis: A geographical hypothesis. *Medical Hypotheses,* Vol.49, pp.477-486.

Chia, Y., Fowler, C.J. Kamm, M.A., Henry, M.M., Lemieux, M. & Swash, M. (1995). Prevalence of bowel dysfunction in patients with multiple sclerosis and bladder dysfunction. *Journal of Neurology,* Vol.242, No.2, pp.105-108.

Coggrave, M. (2008). Neurogenic continence. Part 3: Bowel management strategies. *British Journal of Nursing,* Vol.47, No.15, pp.962-967.

Coggrave, M., Wiesel, P.H. & Norton, C. (2006). Management of faecal incontinence and constipation in adults with central neurological diseases (Review). *Cochrane Database of Systematic Reviews,* Issue 2, Art. No.: CD002115. DOI: 10.1002/14651858.CD002115.pub3.

Curry, Jr., C.E. & Butler, D.M. (2006). Constipation, In: *Handbook of nonprescription drugs: An interactive approach to self-care,* R.R. Berardi, L.A. Kroon, J.H. McDermott, G.D. Newton, M.A. Oszko, N.G. Popovich, T.L. Remington, C.J. Rollins, L.A. Shimp, & K. J. Tietze, (Eds.), 299-326, American Pharmacists Association., Washington, DC.

DasGupta, R. & Fowler, C.J. (2003). Bladder, bowel and sexual dysfunction in multiple sclerosis: Management strategies. *Drugs,* Vol.63, No.2, pp.153-166.

Di Fabio, R.P., Soderberg, J., Choi, T., Hansen, C.R. & Schapiro, R.T. (1998). Extended outpatient rehabiliataion: Its influence on symptom frequency, fatigue, and functional status for persons with progressive multiple sclerosis. *Archives of Physical Medicine and Rehabilitation,* Vol.79, (February1998), pp.141-146.

Dietary Guidelines for Americans. (2010). Report of the DGAC on the Dietary Guidelines for Americans, 2010. Available from http://.www.cnpp.usda.gov/dgas2010-dgacreport.htm.

Emmanuel A. (2010). Rehabilitation in practice: Managing neurogenic bowel dysfunction. *Clinical Rehabilitation,* Vol.24, pp.483-488.

Frank, L., Kleinman, L., Farup, C., Taylor, L. & Miner Jr., P. (1999). Psychometric validation of a constipation symptom assessment questionnaire. *Scandinavian Journal of Gastroenterology,* Vol.34, pp.870-877.

Gill, K.P., Chia, Y.W., Henry, M.M. & Shorvon, P.J. (1994). Defecography in multiple sclerosis patients with severe constipation. *Radiology,* Vol.191, No.2, pp.553-556.

Goodin, D.S. (2010). The genetic basis of multiple sclerosis: A model for MS susceptibility. *Neurology,* Vol.10, No.101, Available from: http://www.biomedcentral.com/1471-2377/10/101.

Goodman, S. & Gulick, E.E. (2008). Dietary practices of people with multiple sclerosis. *International Journal of MS Care,* Vol.10, No.2, pp.47-57.

Gulick, E.E. (2011). Bowel management related quality of life in people with multiple sclerosis: Psychometric evaluation of the QoL-BM measure. *International Journal of Nursing Studies,* Vol.48, pp.1066-1070.

Gulick, E.E. (2010). Comparison of prevalence, related medical history, symptoms, and interventions regarding bowel dysfunction in persons with multiple sclerosis. *Journal of Neuroscience Nursing,* Vol.42, No.4 (August 2010), pp.E12-E23.

Gulick, E.E. (1997). Correlates of quality of life among persons with multiple sclerosis. *Nursing Research,* Vol 46, No.6, pp.305-311.

Gulick, E.E. & Goodman, S. (2006). Physical activity among people with multiple sclerosis. *International Journal of MS Care,* Vol.8, pp.121-129.

Guyton, A.C. & Hall, J.E. (2006). The autonomic nervous system and the adrenal medulla, Propulsion and mixing of food in the alimentary tract, In: *Textbook of medical physiology,* pp.748-760, 781-806, Elsevier & Saunders, Philadellphia, PA.

Hay-Smith, E.J.C., Siegert, R.J., Weatherall, M. & Abernethy, D.A. (2007). Bladder and bowel dysfunction in multiple sclerosis: A review of treatment effectiveness. *Australian and New Zealand Continence Journal,* Vol.13, No. 3, pp.81-89.

Hennessey, A,, Robertson, N.P., Swingler, R. & Compston D.A.S. (1999). Urinary, faecal and sexual dysfunction in patients with multiple sclerosis. *Journal of Neurology,* Vol.246, pp.1027-1032.

Herdon, R.M. (2003). The pathology of multiple sclerosis and its variants. In *Multiple sclerosis: Immunology, pathology, and pathophysiology,* R.M. Herdon (Ed.), 185-197, New York: Demos Medical Publishing, Inc.

Hinds, J.P., Eidelman, B.H. & Wald, A. (1990). Prevalence of bowel dysfunction in multiple sclerosis: A population survey. *Gastroenterology,* Vol.98, pp.1538-1542.

Hinds, J.P. & Wald, A. (1989). Colonic and anorectal dysfunction associated with multiple sclerosis. *The American Journal of Gastroenterology,* Vol.84, No.6, pp.587-595.

Hongisto, S.M., Paajanen, L., Saxelin, M. & Korpela, R. (2006). A combination of fibre-rich rye bread and yoghurt containing Lactobacillus GG improves bowel function in women with self-reported constipation. *European Journal of Clinical Nutrition,* Vol.60, pp.319-324.

Irwin, K. (2003). Back to basics 1: Assessment of bowel dysfunction. *Journal of Community Nursing,* Vol.17, No.11, pp.26-32.

Irwin, K. (2002). Digital rectal examination/manual removal of faeces in adults. *Journal of Community Nursing,* Vol.16, No.4, pp.16-20.

Khan, F., Pallant, J.F., Shea, T.L. & Whishaw, M. (2009). Multiple sclerosis: Prevalence and factors impacting bladder and bowel function in an Australian community cohort. *Disability and Rehabilitation,* Vol.31, No.19, pp.1567-1576.

Koch-Henriksen, N. & Sorensen P.S. (2010). The changing demographic pattern of multiple sclerosis epidemiology. *Lancet Neurology,* Vol.9, No.5, pp.520-532.

Krogh, K. & Christensen, P. (2009). Neurogenic colorectal and pelvic floor dysfunction. *Best Practice & Research Clinical Gastroenterology,* Vol.23, pp.531-543.

Kyle, G. et al. (2005). A procedure for the digital removal of faeces. *Nursing Standard,* Vol.19, No.20, (January 26, 2005), pp.33-39.

Lewicky-Gaupp, C., Morgan, D.M., Chey, W.D., Muellerleile, P. & Fenner D.E. (2008). Successful physical therapy for constipation related to puborectalis dyssynergia improves symptom severity and quality of life. *Diseases of the Colon and Rectum,* Vol.51, (June 27, 2008), pp.1686-1691.

Locke III, G.R., Pemberton, J.H. & Phillips, S.F. (2000). American Gastroenterological Association technical review on constipation. *Gastroenterology,* Vol.119, No.6, pp.1766-1778.

McClurg, D., Hagen, S., Hawkins, S. & Lowe-Strong, A. (2011). Abdominal massage for the alleviation of constipation symptoms in people with multiple sclerosis: A randomized controlled feasibility study. *Multiple Sclerosis Journal,* Vol.17, No.2, pp.223-233.

Mehta, B.K. (2010). New hypotheses on sunlight and the geographic variability of multiple sclerosis prevalence. *Journal of the Neurological Sciences,* Vol.292, pp. 5-10.

Milo, R. & Kahana, E. (2010). Multiple sclerosis: Geoepidemiology, genetics and the environment. *Autoimmunity Reviews,* Vol.9, pp.A387-A394.

Mortensen, N. & Humphreys, M.S. (1991). The anal continence plug: A disposable device for patients with anorectal incontinence. *The Lancet,* Vol.338, (August 3, 1991), pp.295-297.

Moses, Jr., H., Picone, M.A. & Smith, V.C. (2008). *Clinician's primer on multiple sclerosis: An in-depth overview,* Teva Neuroscience,Consensus Medical Communications, Englwood, CO.

Muller-Lissner, S.A. (1988). Effect of wheat bran on weight of stool and gastrointestinal transit time: A meta analysis. *British Medical Journal,* Vol.296, (February 27, 1988), pp.615-617.

Munteis, E., Andreu, M., Martinez-Rodriguez, J.E., Ois, A., Bory, F. & Roquer, J. (2008). Manometric correlations of anorectal dysfunction and biofeedback outcome in patients with multiple sclerosis. *Multiple Sclerosis,* Vol.14, 237-242.

Namey, M.A. & Halper, J (2000). Bowel Disturbance, In: *Multiple sclerosis, diagnosis, management, and rehabilitation,* J.S. Burkes & K.P. Johnson, (Eds.), 453-459, Demos, New York.

Nordenbo, A.M., Andersen, J.R. & Andersen, J.T. (1996). Disturbances of ano- rectal function in multiple sclerosis. *Journal of Neurology,* Vol.243, pp.445-451.

Norton, C. & Chelvanayagam, S. (2010). Bowel problems and coping strategies in people with multiple sclerosis. *British Journal of Nursing,* Vol.19, No.4, pp.220-226.

Norton, C. & Kamm, M.A. (1999). Outcome of biofeedback for faecal incontinence. *British Journal of Surgery,* Vol.86, pp.1159-1163.

Nortvedt, M.W., Riise, T., Frugard, J., Mohn, J., Bakke, A., Skar, A.B., Nyland, H., Glad, S.B. & Myhr, K.M. (2007). Prevalence of bladder, bowel and sexual problems among multiple sclerosis patients two to five years after diagnosis. *Multiple Sclerosis,* Vol.13, pp.106-112.

Pellatt, G.C. (2007). Clinical skills: Bowel elimination and management of complications. *British Journal of Nursing,* Vol.16, No.6, pp.351-355.

Petajan, J.H., Gappmaier, E., White, A.T., Spencer, M.K., Mino, L. & Hicks, R.W. (1996). Impact of aerobic training on fitness and quality of life in multiple sclerosis. *Annals of Neurology,* Vol.39, pp.432-441.

Petajan, J.H. & White, A.T. (1999). Recommendations for physical activity in patients with multiple sclerosis. *Sports Medicine,* Vol.27, No.3, pp.179- 191.

Pierce, E., Cowan, P. & Stokes, M. (2001). Managing faecal retention and incontinence in neurodisability. *British Journal of Nursing,* Vol.10, No.9, pp.592-601.

Powell, M. & Rigby, D. (2000). Management of bowel dysfunction: Evacuation difficulties. *Nursing Standard,* Vol.4, No.47, (August 9, 2000), pp.47-51.

Rao, S.S.C. (2007). Constipation: Evaluation and treatment of colonic and anorectal motility disorders. *Gastroenterology Clinics of North America,* Vol.36, No.3, pp.687-711.

Rao, S.S.C., Tuteja, A.K., Vellema, T., Kempf, J. & Stessman, M. (2004). Dyssynergic defecation: Demographics, symptoms, stool patterns, and quality of life. *Journal of Clinical Gastroenterology,* Vol.38, No.8, (September 2004), pp.680-685.

Rigby, D. & Powell M. (2005). Causes of constipation and treatment options. *Primary Health Care,* Vol.15, No.2, (March 2005), pp.41-50.

Ringel, Y. (2003). Measuring colonic transit time. *Medscape Gastroenterology,* Vol. 5, No.2, pp.1-2, Available from, www.medscape.com/viewarticle/463895.

Shariati, A., Maceda, J.S. & Hale, D.S. (2008). High-fiber diet for treatment of constipation in women with pelvic floor disorders. *Obstetrics & Gynecology,* Vol.111, No.4, (April 2008), pp.908-913.

Sicherer, S.H. (2011). Epidemiology of food allergy. *Journal of Allergy and Clinical Immunology,* Vol.127, pp.594-602.

Slappendel, R., Simpson, K., Dubois, D. & Keininger, D.L. (2006). Validation of the PAC-SYM questionnaire for opioid-induced constipation in patients with chronic low back pain. *European Journal of Pain,* Vol. 10, pp.209-217.

Slater, W. (2003). Management of faecal incontinence of a patient with spinal cord injury. *British Journal of Nursing,* Vol.12, No.12, pp.727-734.

Sloka, S., Silva, C., Pryse-Phillips, W., Patten, S., Metz, L. & Wee Yong, V. (2011). A Quantitative analysis of suspected environmental causes of MS. *Canadian Journal of Neurological Sciences,* Vol.38, pp.98-105.

Soni, A. (2007). Screening colonoscopy among U.S. noninstitutionalized adult population age 50 and older, 2005. Agency for Healthcare Research and Quality, (November 2007).

Sorensen, M., Lorentzen, M., Petersen, J. & Christiansen, J. (1991). Anorectal dysfunction in patients with urologic disturbance due to multiple sclerosis. *Diseases of the Colon and Rectum,* Vol.34, pp.136-139.

Swash, M., Snooks, S.J. & Chalmers, D.H.K. (1987). Parity as a factor in incontinence in multiple sclerosis. *Archives of Neurology,* Vol.44, (May 1987), pp.504-508.

Tjandra, J.J., Chan, M.K.Y., Hung Yeh, C. & Murray-Green, C. (2008). Sacral nerve stimulation is more effective than optimal medical therapy for severe fecal incontinence: A randomized, controlled study. *Diseases of the Colon & Rectum,* Vol.51, pp.494-502.

Vaizey, C.J., Carapeti, E, Cahill, J.A. & Kamm, M.A. (1999). Prospective comparison of faecal incontinence grading systems. *Gut,* Vol.44, pp.77- 80.

Vollmer, T.L., Ni, W., Stanton, S. & Hadjimichael, O. (1999). The NARCOMS patient registry: A resource for investigators. *International Journal of MS Care,* Vol 1, No.1, (September 1999), pp.12-15.

Vukusic S. & Confavreux, C. (2007). Natural history of multiple sclerosis: Risk factors and prognostic indicators. *Current Opinion in Neurology,* Vol.20, pp.269-274.

Wald, A. (1986). Colonic transit and anorectal manometry in chronic idiopathic constipation. *Archives of Internal Medicine,* Vol.146, (September 1986), pp.1713-1716.

Wald, A. (2007). Appropriate use of laxatives in the management of constipation. *Current Gastroenterology Reports,* Vol.9, pp.410-414.

Waldron, D.J., Horgan, P.G., Patel, F.R., Maguire R. & Given H. F. (1993). Multiple sclerosis: Assessment of colonic and anorectal function in the presence of faecal incontinence. *International Journal of Colorectal Diseases,* Vol.8, pp.220-224.

Walker, P.C. (2006). Diarrhea, In: *Handbook of nonprescription drugs: An interactive approach to self-care,* R.R. Berardi, L.A. Kroon, J.H. McDermott, G.D. Newton, M.A. Oszko, N.G. Popovich, T.L. Remington, C.J. Rollins, L.A. Shimp, & K. J. Tietze, (Eds.), 327--350, American Pharmacists Association. Washington, DC.

Weber, J., Grise, P., Roquebert, M., Hellot, M.F., Mihout, B., Samson, M., Beuret-Blanquart, F., Pasquis, P. & Denis, P. (1987). Radiopague markers transit and anorectal manometry in 16 patients with multiple sclerosis and urinary bladder dysfunction. *Diseases of the Colon and Rectum,* Vol.30, pp.95-100.

Weinshenker, B.G. (1993). The natural history of multiple sclerosis. *Multiple Sclerosis,* Vol.1, No.1, pp.2-3.

Weinshenker, B.G. (1998). The natural history of multiple sclerosis: Update 1998. *Seminars in Neurology,* Vol.18, No.3, pp.301-307.

Whiteley, J. (2007). The effects of urinary and faecal incontinence on the skin. *Journal of Community Nursing,* Vol.21, No.10, pp.26-30.

Wiesel, P.H., Norton C., Glickman, S & Kamm, M.A. (2001). Pathophysiology and management of bowel dysfunction in multiple sclerosis. *European Journal of Gastroenterology & Hepatology,* Vol.13, pp.441-448.

Wiesel, P.H., Norton, C., Roy, A.J., Storrie, J.B., Bowers, J. & Kamm, M.A. (2000). Gut focused behavioural treatment (biofeedback) for constipation and faecal incontinence in multiple sclerosis. *Journal of Neurological and Neurosurgical Psychiatry,* Vol. 69, pp.240-243.

Willer, C.J., Dyment D.A., Risch, N.J., Sadovonick, A.D. & Ebers, G.C. (2003). Twin concordance and sibling recurrence rates in multiple sclerosis. *Proceedings of the National Academy of Sciences of the USA,* Vol.100, No.22, (October 28, 2003), pp.12877-12882.

Wollin W., Bennie, M., Leech, C., Windsor, C. & Spencer, N. (2005). Multiple sclerosis and continence issues: An exploratory study. *British Journal of Nursing,* Vol.14, No.8, pp.439-446.

10

Multimodal Treatment of Constipation: Surgery, Rehabilitation or Both?

Luigi Brusciano et al.*
XI Division of General and Obesity Surgery, Master in Coloproctology, Second University of Naples Italy

1. Introduction

Constipation accounts for 20% in western world population. In absence of any organic aetiology, this disorder may be related to bad alimentary habits based on inadequate introduction of the three components of stool (fibres, probiotics and water) that are essential for the physiologic activity of colon. Chronic constipation may be also associated with either colic or rectal anatomo-functional alterations. Colonic constipation (slow transit constipation) is usually related to a motility disorder (inertia coli) associated with a reduction of propagating contraction waves and decreased Cajal' cells; on the other hand, rectal outlet dysfunction type constipation may be related to anatomical alterations (e.g. internal mucosal prolapse, rectocele) causing difficult rectal outlet and functional pelviperineal dyssynergia. The physiologic defaecatory act involves not only synchronism between rectum and anus, but even correct thoraco-abdominoperineal dynamics and vertebral position. This has to be carefully assessed by considering patient's ability to accomplish adequate thoraco-abdominoperineal muscle movements needed for both adequate defaecatory dynamics and urine and stool retention. Therefore, the ideal treatment should not only address anatomical alterations such as mucosal prolapse, rectocele, rectorectal intussusception and sphincter defects, usually requiring a surgical approach, but even functional disorders, often insidious and difficult to detect. Surgery is mandatory to treat pathological findings, that physically represent an obstacle to fecal transit in the rectum. Many surgical techniques have been developed for the treatment of outlet obstruction with conflicting results. STARR (stapled transanal rectal resection) is a new surgical procedure that was launched by Longo in 2001. It is a minimally invasive transanal operation for rectocele and mucosal/rectal prolapse using a double circular stapler. This procedure is indicated when rectal mucosal prolapse is thought to be the cause of difficult defecation, and appears to be a rational treatment. This treatment aims to normalize the anatomical relationship of the anal mucosa with hemorrhoidal piles and anal sphincters by restoring the prolapse and improving venous perfusion. The procedure pulls the anal

---

* Crescenzo Di Stazio, Paolo Limongelli, Gian Mattia Del Genio, Salvatore Tolone, Saverio Sansone, Francesco Lucido, Ignazio Verde, Antonio D'Alessandro, Roberto Ruggiero, Simona Gili, Assia Topatino, Vincenzo Amoroso, Pina Casalino, Giovanni Docimo and Ludovico Docimo
XI Division of General and Obesity Surgery. Master in Coloproctology. Second University of Naples, Italy

mucosa and perianal tissues upwards and decreases the friction and impact on the tissue surface, which is a cause of difficult defecation. In the mechanism of defecation, the movement associated with the anal sphincters is triggered by the sensory perception on the anal mucosa and anal skin. If the physiological functions of all the involved organs are under optimal conditions, then the mucosa and sphincters can maintain the normal anatomical relationshiep. In January 2006, the European STARR registry was initiated. According to the results published in 2009 on 2838 patients, the improvement in rectal function and quality of life was statistically significant. A multicenter study conducted in Spain between 2001 and 2006 concluded that this procedure is associated with low morbidity and short hospital stay and is an effective treatment option for obstructed defecation syndrome. According to a Milan study reported in 2008, STARR is safe and effective in the treatment of solitary rectal ulcer associated with internal rectal prolapse and has minimal complications and no recurrence after 2 years (Boccasanta et al., 2008). After operation functional outcome shows an improvement in defecation with reduction of the mean Constipation Score. Less pain during evacuation was reported by patients, also as a consequence of reduced pushing to defecate and reduced use of digital assistance. The frequency of complete defecation was increased, so the patient's satisfaction was favorable. Anorectal manometry reveals decrease in the maximum resting and squeezing pressure of the anal canal and in rectal compliance until one month after the operation, compared with the preoperative levels, but they recovered to preoperative levels at 6 months after the operation. This effect is probably the consequence of the anal stretching during operation. Patients show increase in basal sphincter pressure and maximal squeeze pressure, probably for the absence of inhibition that was acted by redundant rectal mucosa on the transitional zone. Recently, a new device the CCS-30 Contour Transtarr was developed by the same Professor Longo. A multicenter prospective study from Naples confirms that the device is effective and safe and has functional results similar to those of the conventional STARR (Renzi et al., 2008). This procedure (with both techniques), according to most authors, is effective; the postoperative pain is mild, and the procedure is very much accepted among colorectal surgeons for the treatment of rectocele as well as for internal rectal prolapse in patients with obstructed defecation. Yet, it should be emphasized that STARR is associated with complications such as postoperative bleeding, chronic proctalgia, rectovaginal fistula, stricture, and fecal incontinence (Gagliardi et al., 2008). Some of these are "learning curve" complications and can be avoided instead many authors stress that if this procedure is performed in selected cases by skilled specialists, most complications can be avoided. The use of an anastomotic stapler has been reported to result in a higher rate of anastomotic stricture formation. However, staples applied to the lower mucosal layer with few connecting tissues are eliminated during a short time, and do not form granuloma that might induce stenosis. In patients with enterocele and puborectalis dyssynergia, this procedure is contraindicated (unless the enterocele is repaired simultaneously on laparoscopy). In view of conflicting reports on the safety and efficacy of the STARR procedure, a European group of experts was founded in October 2006; and in June 2008, following a consensus conference with evidence-based conclusions, they published guidelines on inclusion and exclusion criteria as well as a diagnostic and therapeutic algorithm for the STARR procedure in ODS. These recommendations were based on the experience of 11 specialists in coloproctology and pelvic floor disease, pioneers in the STARR procedure, and it was concluded after a 100% consensus within the group. It was also concluded that this procedure can be performed with either of the devices, depending on the size of the prolapsed or rectocele and on the personal experience of the surgeon. Patient selection is crucial, as is the use of the standardized diagnostic and therapeutic approach. A considerable example of this is given by the study of Zehler that compared functional and clinical short and long-term outcome after stapled transanal rectal resection and found results after 1 year comparable with the functional outcome even after 5 years. The median clinical score improved significantly already after 1 year in these patients and remained stable at 5-year follow-up. In contrast, those patients who failed treatment showing no improvement in the short term, remained symptomatic without improvement in OOS and SSS scores. Eighty per cent of the patients were still satisfied. The author concludes that short-term improvement after STARR predicts long-term outcome in obstructed defecation syndrome caused by a rectocele. The reason of such findings is probably the unaccomplished diagnosis of the disease with an omission of the functional aspect of the trouble. In those patients showing poor outcome, or unstable with time, the functional disturbance was probably prevalent compared to anatomical; diagnosis missed this aspect and consequently treatment was inadequate. Pelviperineal dyssynergia is a functional alteration, characterized by absence of puborectalis muscle relaxation, and inability to relax pelvic floor during attempted defecation. This can cause a delay of rectal stool transit, so that the rectum itself reabsorbs water and stools become harder, drier and difficult to evacuate. Clinically, this can result in painful effort, bleeding after defecation, long periods spent in bathroom, digitation, and sense of incomplete evacuation. In the long term patient may develop reduction of rectal sensitivity with larger volumes of faeces required to feel the need to evacuate (Brusciano et al., 2009). The frequent presence of concurrent alterations (anatomical and functional) causing the symptoms is the explanation of worse results than expected after treatment. This is particularly frequent in those with a thoraco-abdomino-perineal dyssynergia not adequately recognized and simultaneously treated. Supporting this theory Rao showed that systematically assessing anorectal physiology in patients with defecation disorders revealed new information in 88% of patients that led to a change in the management in 76% of cases. Pelviperineal rehabilitation, that teaches patients how to relax pelvic floor muscles, has showed good results by treating the functional aspect of pelvic floor disorders. Nowadays treatment comprises a series of rehabilitation techniques as physiokinesitherapy, biofeedback, electrostimulation and volumetric rehabilitation. Previously published studies reporting on the use of rehabilitation techniques such as biofeedback, muscular training and electrostimulation, have showed a success rate ranging between 47% and 100%. There is lack of agreement on a standard test to select patients who may benefit from such treatment. Particularly, although a clinical and instrumental work-up is commonly carried out by proctologists to characterize these patients, physiatric assessment is not thoroughly accomplished. To correctly approach the problem each aspect of pathology must be detected and specifically treated, with surgery (when anatomical), rehabilitation (when functional) or both (when associated). While the anatomical aspect of the problem is commonly detected by standard clinical and instrumental work-up associated functional disorders are often neglected. A diagnostic protocol, including the evaluation of either physiatric or instrumental findings, has been previously reported by our group to identify patients amenable for pelviperineal rehabilitation treatment (Brusciano et al., 2007). The protocol is based on proctologic examination, clinico-physiatric assessment (puborectalis contraction, pubococcygeal test, perineal defence reflex, muscular synergies, postural examination) and instrumental evaluation (anorectal manometry, anal US and dynamic defaecography).

2. Diagnostic protocol

Clinical and functional evaluation was based on the analysis of the following parameters:

Puborectalis relaxation (relaxation pattern), searching for a paradox muscle's contraction and absence or incomplete relaxation, by rectal examination.

Pubococcygeal (PC) test (puborectalis contraction pattern) evaluating either the phasic contraction, subjectively classified as good, moderate or fair, or the tonic contraction by asking patient to contract the anus, for the longest period of time (classified as good when >9 sec; moderate when ranging between 2 and 9 sec; or fair when < 2sec). The muscular fatigue is also assessed by asking patient to contract the anus as many times as possible for at least 5 seconds, and to rest for 10 sec (classifying it as good when more then 9 times; moderate when ranging between 2 and 9 times; fair when <less than 2 times).

Perineal defence reflex consisted in the assessment of pelvic floor and abdominal muscles' action, following an intra-abdominal pressure's increase. Patient is asked to cough, so that the physician can notice the perineal muscles' contraction, resulting either in a physiological rising (reflex present) or a pathological descending (reflex absent) that, if marked, can be associated with emission of urine and flatulence.

Muscular synergyes, i.e. the activity of both agonist (glutei and abductors) and antagonist muscles (abdominals, diaphragm), were evaluated in Sims' position by asking the patient to contract the anus, after placing a hand over the abdominal wall while observing gluteus and abductor contraction.

Muscle synergy was defined as agonist, by the simultaneous contraction of anus and either glutei or abductors, whereas antagonist by the simultaneous contraction of anus and abdominal muscle.

Postural examination was based on the evaluation of lumbar lordosis by using a "plumb line". This is a straight line formed by a string attached to a hanging weight. It establishes a vertical line which is straight up and down the spine. The distance between the "plumb line" and the spinous process of L3 is measured by a ruler considering a range between 25 and 35 mm as normal.

2.1 Instrumental assessment

Anorectal manometry evaluated a series of distinct parameters:

anal resting pressure (ARP) (normal value between 55 and 75 mmHg; hypertonic if > 75 mmHg; hypotonic if < 50 mmHg);

maximal voluntary contraction (MCV) (amplitude normal value if > 120 mmHg; duration normal value if > 22 sec);

rectal sensory included conscious rectal sensory threshold (CRST) (normal value 25-45 ml), and maximum tolerated volume (MCV) (normal value 80-160 ml) , defining either hyposensitivity (MTV > 160 or CRST > 40) or hypersensitivity (CRST < 40);

rectoanal inhibitory reflex (RAIR) by considering both the percentage of relaxation (normal values ≥ 85%) and the balloon expulsion test (the balloon was filled up with air until the subject reported desire to defecate: the ballon was considered not expelled if the time required by the patient overcame 1 minute).

Defaecography evaluated the pelvic floor descent. This was defined as the vertical distance between the pubococcygeal line and the ano-rectal junction in straining (expressed in millimetres) A distance greater than 4 cm was considered as pathologic perineal descent.

Anal ultrasonography assessed the puborectalis relaxation. The absence of relaxation of the puborectalis muscle was defined when no increase of the distance between the inner edge of the muscle posteriorly and the probe measured at rest and on straining was detectable. In female patients the puborectalis relaxation was also evaluated by vaginal US that leaves the puborectalis sling relatively undisturbed and therefore more free to relax.

To assess potential implications of these parameters, considered responsible of constipation, in the functional aspects of these disorders we compared them in a large number of patients with constipation and incontinence as well as in healthy controls.

Several altered parameters were identified in patients with constipation or incontinence compared to HC demonstrating strong correlations between physiatric disorders and the symptoms.

We, moreover, recently performed further studies that show how successful specific treatment of the physiatric disorders, in patients with altered physiatric parameters, improves proctologic symptoms.

These results allow to suppose a causal relationship between physiatric parameters, functional alteration and clinical symptoms.

A rehabilitation scheme based on different techniques (biofeedback, electrostimulation, physiokinesitherapy, and volumetric rehabilitation) should seek to correct those functional alterations. For instance, the finding of lumbar lordosis needs to be treated by postural physiokinesitherapy, whereas the absence of perineal defense reflex needs physiokinesitherapy to synchronize the muscular function of the thoracic, abdominal, and pelviperineal muscle district. On the other hand, an absence of puborectalis muscle relaxation and a decrease in the maximum voluntary contraction of external anal sphincter should be managed by biofeedback and electrostimulation therapy.

Another example, in the case of a constipated patient with a rectocele, and with concurrent abnormal rectal sensation or non-relaxing puborectalis muscle on straining and alteration of recto anal inhibitory reflex (RAIR), although surgical correction will improve rectal emptying, therapy could not be considered appropriate without addressing the functional component of the syndrome.

Similarly, the mere treatment of the functional disorders without correcting anatomical alteration is a sketchy therapy. Concerning this, we also assessed the outcome of rehabilitation treatment, using the rehabilitation diagnostic protocol, in patients with or without previous surgery for rectal outlet obstruction.

All patients selected for rehabilitation treatment were divided into two groups:

group A consisted of patients with rectal outlet obstruction never submitted to previous surgical treatment;

group B consisted of patients operated of STARR procedure for rectal outlet obtruction (with a rectocele > 4 cm, rectal internal mucosal prolapse, and recto-rectal and recto-anal intussusceptions).

We observed in both groups significant improvement of physiatric parameters while operated patients showed better clinical outcome at six months follow-up. These results support the theory of a multifactorial pathogenesis of such disorders and show that specific treatment of different components causing the same symptoms is the best approach with the best outcome.

3. Pelvi-perineal rehabilitation programme

Patients were offered one session of treatment, lasting an average of 45 minutes, every 5 days for a minimum of 10-12 overall sessions. The rehabilitation treatment aims to correct the thoraco-abdomino-perineal dyssinergia by using different means as physiokinesytherapy (by operator's hands), biofeedback and electrostimulation (by specific probes) and volumetric rehabilitation (by enema). Although the sequential use of these different tools may differ among patients, all techniques are indispensable for a thorough rehabilitation treatment as following described. Firstly, patients were informed on the anatomical and physiological principles of pelvic floor district, stressing on the importance of the re-educational aspect of rehabilitation. Thus, patients should be knowledged in terms of anatomical and physiological notions on which body area is to be treated, in order to best interact during rehabilitation. By performing anal and/or vaginal digital exploration, physician highlights puborectalis anatomical position, inviting patients either to pushing out or squeezing to respectively simulate evacuation or stool retention. Moreover, patients were informed about the role of thoraco-abdominal and perineal muscles districts, whose synergy is determinant for an adequate defaecation act; one way to let patient learn this harmony between thoraco-abdominal-perineal districts is to show the distinction between thoracic and abdominal breathing. Rehabilitation treatment was based on four different techniques:

1. Physiokinesitherapy, obtained throughout thoraco-abdomino-perineal muscles coordination training, as previously described. According to Bourdiol-Bortolin technique, patients were taught to direct propulsive force into the pelvis by taking a deep breath, contracting the upper abdominal and diaphragmatic muscles (diaphragmatic breathing exercises), and simultaneously relaxing and protruding the lower abdomen. A visible protrusion of the latter, indicated a correct performance. Unlike other rehabilitation techniques specifically focused on pelvic floor dyssinergia, physiokinesotherapy aims to treat postural defects and limitation of hips motion as well as improve respiratory dynamics required for the stability of thoraco-abdominal and perineal muscles districts. The need for such a treatment have to be highlighted with a general evaluation (while often attention is focused on pelvic district) to identify postural defects, articular blocks (specially lumbo-sacral) or anomaly in respiratory dynamics.

2. external electrical stimulation was used to help patients to be conscious of the perineal district and then improve its muscles performance. It was performed using an anal probe with pulse generator (Pelveen Care, Coloplast, Bologna Italia). Indeed, an adequate electrical stimulation method, along with standard values of different parameters, have not yet been determined in patients with defaecatory disorders. Prior to therapy the electrical stimulation level fit for each patient, was evaluated by fixing it just below the point where

patient started to feel either discomfort or pain. Stimulation therapy was performed once a day, for 20 min over 10–12 sessions either at outpatient clinic or home.

3. Biofeedback (BFT) was performed using the electromyographic (EMG) biofeedback system (Pelveen Care, Coloplast, Bologna Italy). The visual feedback was provided by observing changes in pressure activity on a monitor screen. The patients were taught to practice mainly contraction and relaxation manoeuvres of the anal canal, meanwhile evaluating the activity of abdominal muscles or glutei/abductors muscles, by using the surface electromyography. Each session lasted 30–50 min over 10–14 sessions.

4. The principles of volumetric rehabilitation (VR) are based on the mechanical distension of the rectum (enema)

The aim of this technique is to restore the impaired rectal sensation. The technique involves the administration, twice daily, of a tepid water enema. The initial volume equals the manometric maximum tolerated volume (MTV) or conscious rectal sensitivity threshold (CRST) on the basis of the underlined defaecatory disorders. The subject is asked to hold the liquid after perceiving it in the rectum, by strongly contracting the anus for no more than 30 seconds. The last step is to expel the water through a relaxation of the pelvic floor and an effective abdominal straining. The goal of this rehabilitation technique is to let patient understand the three basic phases of the defaecatory act (perception; retaining; passing), in order to become aware of the pelviperineal muscolar activity. Thus, patients may improve their own rectal sensibility. Patients are instructed to self-administer the enemas at home.

4. Results

In our study the diagnostic protocol revealed abnormal values in symptomatic patients compared to Healthy Controls. Particularly they showed significantly higher values of lumbar lordosis values as well as lower rate in the presence of both perineal defence reflex and puborectalis relaxation. Furthermore patients performed a worse PC tests and showed a higher rate of muscle synergies presence (either agonist or antagonist) as compared to controls. Instrumental diagnostic examination also evidenced important differences between groups for all analyzed parameters; both manometric and defecographic patterns resulted pathologically skewed in terms of values or percentage comparing patients with Healthy Controls. Rehabilitation treatment acted positively on symptoms and exerted a tangible action on all evaluated clinical-instrumental parameters. Along with the Wexner score, all clinico-physiatric parameters (lumbar lordosis, perineal defence reflex, pubo-rectalis relaxation, PC test and agonist and antagonist muscular synergies) significantly improved after treatment. Some parameters received a particularly positive influence by rehabilitation: correction of lumbar lordosis was rapidly achieved with restoration of physiologic posture by means of physiatric exercises and this allows to reach a correct extension of pubo-rectalis muscle and, consequently, a better function with an improved grade of relaxation. Also Pubococcygeal (PC) test (puborectalis contraction pattern) recorded a great improvement after treatment, both about the entity than about the duration of contraction and the muscular fatigue. This effect is clearly consequence of muscular exercise, as for any other skeletal muscle, and is associated to hypertrophy. For the same reason this effect is strictly dependent by exercise and in the long term, with a reduction of interest by patient, it tends to decrease. To the contrary improvement of agonist antagonist muscular synergies tends to be stable with time; rehabilitation produced a strong impact on this parameter by teaching patients to correctly recruit muscles involved in one action and to selectively relax those opponents. This learned pattern of muscular contraction and relaxation involves many different anatomical structure, and his target is the instauration of an harmonic interaction between thoracic abdominal and pelvic districts. Clinical improvements reflexes on instrumental findings; particularly manometrics parameters showing positive modification were anal resting pressure, rectal sensation, recto-anal inhibitory reflex and duration of MCV, and balloon expulsion test. Those are expression of muscular reinforcement and coordination but also of sensitive improvement and consciousness. Finally both groups showed improvement in PAC-QOL after rehabilitation treatment. Scanty reports have been published in literature regarding the assessment of patients affected by rectal outlet obstruction and amenable for pelviperineal rehabilitation treatment. Our results seem to justify the need for conducting in patients with defaecatory disorders, an extensive diagnostic protocol based on the evaluation of 14 different parameters aiming to identify muscle dyssynergia. In our opinion, it would not seem fair to select patients on the basis of a single modified parameter (e.g. absence of puborectalis muscle relaxation) as usually reported by the majority of proctologists, whereas a thorough pre-treatment study protocol may help to better understand the physiopathologic mechanisms underlying each patient's clinical picture and to predict the impact of rehabilitation on outcome. The frequent finding of anatomical alterations in patients with constipation is probably the reason of the great rate of unrecognized functional disorders. Those anatomical abnormality are commonly considered the only responsible of symptoms and often the therapy is focused selectively on their correction with a complete omission of functional aspects also composing the clinical picture. Consequently surgical therapy of such a patient will be only a partial correction of the problem, with incomplete resolution of symptoms and predisposing to recurrence. A systematic evaluation of those patients, with particular attention to functional patterns, should be considered as a routine diagnostic protocol to clearly understand each aspect of the pathology and to allow a tailored surgical, rehabilitative or combined treatment.

5. References

Boccasanta P, Venturi M, Calabro G, Maccioco M, Roviaro GC. *Stapled transanal rectal resection in solitary rectal ulcer associated with prolaps of the rectum: a prospective study. Dis Colon Rectum* 2008; 51: 348-54.

Brusciano L, Limongelli P, Del Genio G, Rossetti G, Sansone S, Healey A, Maffettone V, Napolitano V, Pizza F, Tolone S, Del Genio A. *Clinical and instrumental parameters in patients with constipation and incontinence: their potential implications in the functional aspects of these disorders.* Int J Colorectal Dis 2009; 24: 961-967.

Brusciano L, Limongelli P, del Genio G, Sansone S, Rossetti G, Maffettone V, Napolitano V, Sagnelli C, Pizza F, del Genio A. *Useful parameters helping proctologists to identify patients with defaecatory disorders that may be treated with pelvic floor rehabilitation.* Tech Coloproctol. 2007 11:45–50

Gagliardi G, Pescatori M, Altomare DF, et al. *Results, outcome, predictors and complications after stapled transanal resection for obstructed defecation. Dis Colon Rectum* 2008; 51: 186-95.

Renzi A, Talento P, Giardiello C et al. *Stapled transanal rectal resection by a new dedicated device for the surgical treatment of obstructed defecation syndrome caused by rectal intussusaption and rectocele: early results of a multicenter prospective study. Int J Colorectal Dis* 2008; 23: 999-1005

11

Core Aspects of Clinical Development and Trials in Chronic Idiopathic Constipation

M. Scott Harris and Oranee T. Daniels
Georgetown University School of Medicine and Theravance, Inc.
USA

1. Introduction

Chronic constipation is one of the most common conditions, with prevalence by various estimates ranging from 1.9% to 27.2% in the American population (Bharucha et al., 2000; Higgins & Johanson, 2004; Shah et al., 2008). Treatment options range from older over-the-counter laxatives to recently approved prescription drug therapies (Longstreth et al., 2006; Motola et al., 2002; Ramkumar & Rao, 2005; Tack & Müller-Lissner, 2009; Tack et al., 2011; Tramonte et al., 1997). It has been estimated that 6 million to 8.5 million patients seek medical care for constipation each year. Over 70% of these individuals express dissatisfaction with prior medications, pointing to the need for new therapies (Johanson & Kralstein, 2007).

Drugs that have been recently approved or which are in late-stage trials for treatment of constipation are listed in Table 1. These include prokinetic agents (5-HT_4 receptor agonists),

Drug class	Agent	Mechanism of action	Status
5-HT_4 receptor agonist	Prucalopride	Prokinetic: Stimulation of colonic peristalsis	Approved in Europe and Switzerland
	Velusetrag		Completed Phase 2
	Naronapride		Completed Phase 2
Secretagogue	Lubiprostone	ClC2 channel and CFTR channel activator	Approved in US and Switzerland for CIC and IBS-c
	Linaclotide	GCCR agonist	Phase 3 completed in US and Europe
	Plecanatide	GCCR agonist	Phase 2 in US
	A3309	IBAT inhibitor	Phase 2 completed
Absorption inhibitor	Na-H exchange inhibitor	RDX-5791	Phase 2 in US

Table 1. Drugs recently approved or in late-stage clinical trials for chronic idiopathic constipation

secretagogues (guanylate cyclase C receptor agonists, bile acid transport inhibitors, Cl channel activators), and Na-H exchange inhibitors. Prokinetic agents promote colonic motor activity and propulsion, while secretagogues and Na-H exchange inhibitors either induce secretion of water and electrolytes or inhibit their absorption, resulting in more water in luminal contents. All of these agents appear to accelerate colonic transit time and accentuate stool output. There is little known at this point regarding comparative efficacy and safety between individual drugs or drug classes. Although speculative, it is likely that different drugs and drug classes will be used concomitantly in patients who fail to achieve the desired therapeutic response.

Serotonin (5-hydroxytryptamine, 5-HT) is a critical regulator of gastrointestinal motility, sensitivity, and secretion (Gershon, 2004). 5-HT triggers and coordinates intestinal peristalsis through 5-HT_4 receptors expressed mainly on enteric neurons (Gershon & Tack, 2007). The safety of the 5-HT_4 subclass has been brought into scrutiny because of the withdrawal of two previously marketed drugs, as will be discussed below. The highly selective 5-HT_4 agonists currently under development are expected to exhibit more favorable safety profiles with low potential for cardiovascular side effects (DeMaeyer et al., 2008).

This review will provide an oversight of drugs that have been recently approved or are currently in late-stage clinical development for chronic idiopathic constipation (CIC). We will focus on methodologies (endpoints, study populations, biomarkers) that have been employed in proof-of-concept (Phase 2) and late-stage confirmatory clinical trials (Phase 3). We will discuss specific drug properties (dosing, drug-drug interactions, and specificity) that are the expected outcome of these trials. The goal of the clinical development program in CIC is to thoroughly document a drug profile with an acceptable balance between efficacy and safety.

The use of opioids and the side effects of opioid use have reached near epidemic proportions in the United States. The prevalence of constipation in this population is estimated to range between 20% and 70% (Bell et al., 2009; Brown et al., 2006; Kalso et al., 2004). While there have been considerable efforts directed towards the development of drugs for treating opioid-induced constipation, our review will focus on constipation from other causes.

2. Drug properties impacting clinical development

2.1 Pharmacokinetic and pharmacodynamic profiles

Compounds currently in clinical development are intended to be used as chronic oral therapies rather than periodically as rescue treatment. Therefore, pharmacokinetics of each compound after repeated dosing will play an important role in differentiating ease of use (i.e., once daily), potential accumulation, drug-drug interaction, etc. Drugs that promote more frequent and complete defecation may act locally on the GI mucosa or exert their effects systemically. The degree in which systemic exposure drives clinical efficacy varies by drug class, expected site of action in GI tract, and pharmacokinetics of each compound. High molecular weight (e.g., peptides) ordinarily renders a drug non-absorbable. Some constipation drugs have been postulated to exert their effects by local and systemic mechanisms simultaneously (Hoffman et al., 2010). 5-HT_4 agonists currently under development are small molecules that are absorbed and systemically available, while the newer secretagogues, such as linaclotide and plecanatide, are peptides that are unabsorbed and systemically inert (Harris & Cromwell, 2007; Shailubhai et al., 2010). The maximal tolerated dose (MTD) of a systemically available drug depends on many factors, including end-organ toxicities and drug interactions, while the therapeutic limit of non- or minimally absorbed drugs mainly reflects GI tolerance. Irrespective of these considerations, all compounds for the treatment of constipation possess the inherent potential to produce diarrhea when administered at sufficient doses, due presumably to their exaggerated pharmacology rather than some off-target activity. Diarrhea led to study discontinuation in almost 5% of subjects in recent Phase 3 trials of linaclotide (Lembo et al., 2010a).

Absence of systemic exposure minimizes but does not eliminate the possibility drug-drug interactions or drug toxicity. Drug interactions, for example, could still occur with efflux proteins (e.g., p-glycoprotein) at the enterocyte brush border (Huang & Woodcock, 2009). A3309, a non-absorbed inhibitor of bile acid transport (IBAT) that blocks bile acid re-absorption by the terminal ileum (Chey et al., 2011a) could theoretically impair long-term fat-soluble vitamin absorption (Vitamin A, E, D) or lead to other nutritional deficiencies. The choleretic compound class has also been associated with higher rates of abdominal cramping and diarrhea in clinical trials (Odynsi-Shiyanbade et al., 2010).

There have been few examples of non-GI adverse events using the newer 5-HT_4 agonists. As will be discussed below, the infrequency of these events probably relates to higher specificity for the 5-HT_4 receptor than earlier agents. Certain 5-HT_4 agonists (prucalopride and velusetrag) have been associated with a low but increased incidence of headaches and nausea compared with placebo. Although these side effects were reported in smaller percentages of patients in clinical trials of naronapride, the relationship between these adverse events and degree of CNS penetration is unclear (Palme et al., 2010). These side effects have been shown to resolve after the first day of treatment (Camilleri et al., 2008; Goldberg et al., 2010).

Linaclotide is a GCCR agonist and synthetic analog of E. coli ST_a toxin that stimulates intracellular c-GMP activity and active Cl secretion. Linaclotide is released and degraded rapidly in the duodenum (Kessler et al., 2008). This being the case, the stool hydrating effect of linaclotide must rely on a rapid burst of secretion in the upper intestine. Colonic motor dysfunction could potentially blunt or eliminate the subsequent therapeutic responses to linaclotide, reflecting the prodigious organ specific capacity for water reabsorption by the colon, coupled with prolonged transit (Debongnie & Phillips, 1978). Titration of distal stool volume might be difficult to control by a proximally active mechanism, resulting in wider swings in fecal output and higher rates of diarrhea-associated adverse events. Consistent targeting of specific sites along the length of the GI tract could be difficult with a luminally active agent. A 10-fold to 100-fold inter-individual variability in GCC mRNA expression has been observed in the human intestine (Bharucha et al., 2010), adding to the challenge of proper dosing in individual patients.

Plecanatide is a synthetic analogue of naturally occurring uroguanylin that mediates basal secretion and cell volume in humans (Shailubhai et al., 2010). In contrast to linaclotide, which is stabilized by three disulfide bonds that maintain the peptide in a tight configuration (Harris & Cromwell, 2007), the molecular structure of plecanatide contains only two disulfide bonds (Shailubhai et al., 2010), potentially rendering it less stable at its intestinal site of action. Furthermore, its binding to GCC receptors is pH-dependent. Perhaps as a result of these properties, plecanatide manifests three-fold to five-fold lower potency compared with linaclotide in human studies on a concentration basis (Lembo et al., 2010a; Shailubhai et al., 2010). Plecanatide was associated with a lower incidence of diarrhea in a preliminary trial of constipated patients, but this could potentially be representative of lower rates of intestinal secretion induced by the compound (Shailubhai et al., 2010).

2.2 Receptor specificity and off-target effects

5-HT in the GI tract is primarily stored in gut enterochromaffin cells, with a much smaller portion in enteric neurons. High selectivity is an important feature of newer 5-HT_4 agonists like prucalopride, velusetrag, and naronapride. Early 5-HT_4 agonists were associated with non-specific receptor binding and off-target cardiac findings. Metoclopramide, a mixed 5-HT_4 agonist and D_2 antagonist, has been associated with tardive dyskinesia as a result of antagonism of striatal dopamine receptors, leading the FDA to issue a black box warning restricting recommended use (Metozolv Prescribing Information, 2009). Up to 30% of patients using metoclopramide discontinue treatment due to various other CNS side effects (Lee and Kuo, 2010).

Cisapride, a benzamide, was a 5-HT_4 agonist that facilitated release of acetylcholine throughout the gut. It was used widely for treatment of gastro-esophageal reflux disease, gastroparesis and functional dyspepsia (Wiseman & Faulds, 1994). While the efficacy of cisapride in upper gastrointestinal tract motility was widely recognized, its effects on constipation and lower GI motility have been questioned (Abourmarzouk 2011). The loss of effect in the lower GI tract was attributed to concomitant antagonism of the 5-HT_3 and potentially 5-HT_2 receptor, leading to opposing effects on colonic transit and secretion (Masaoka & Tack, 2009).

In 2000, cisapride was withdrawn from the market due to fatal arrhythmias and dose-dependent QT interval prolongation (Masaoka & Tack, 2009). These events occurred notably in patients taking other medications that are known to inhibit the CYP450 3A4 isozyme, e.g., erythromycin, fluconazole and amiodarone. Although the basis of cisapride's arrhythmogenic effect was not fully understood, it has been attributed to blockade of hERG (human ether-a-go-go) potassium channels, and a resulting delay in cardiac action potential repolarization in ventricular muscle and Purkinje fibers, and unrelated to its 5-HT_4 agonist properties (Tonini et al., 1999).

Tegaserod, a 5-HT_4 receptor partial agonist of aminoguanidine indole class, was approved in the United States for the treatment of chronic constipation and irritable bowel syndrome with constipation (Al-Judaibi et al., 2010). Although several studies (Prather et al., 2000; Foxx-Orenstein et al., 2005) demonstrated prokinetic action of tegaserod in both upper and lower GI tract, data regarding improvement of gastric emptying in humans are inconsistent (Talley et al., 2006; Degen et al., 2001, 2005). Tegaserod was withdrawn from the market in 2007 because of a reported numerical imbalance in the number of patients with cardiovascular ischemic adverse events in trials for patients who received tegaserod compared with those on placebo (Pasricha, 2007). Subsequent epidemiologic studies (Anderson et al., 2009; Loughlin et al., 2010) failed to confirm a reported large event differential for tegaserod that was noted incidentally in this clinical trial database.

Tegaserod is now recognized to have significant affinity for non-5-HT_4 receptors, including the 5-HT_{1B}, 5-HT_{1D} and 5-HT_{2B} subtypes (Borman et al., 2002; DeMaeyer et al., 2008). The effects of tegaserod on 5-HT_1 receptors present on blood vessels and platelet aggregation have been implicated as a mechanism accountable for ischemic changes (Chan et al., 2009; DeMaeyer et al., 2008; Serebruany et al., 2010). Moreover, the potent 5-HT_{2B} antagonism of tegaserod has been postulated to counteract its 5-HT_4 prokinetic effect (Borman et al., 2002). Low oral bioavailability (10%) may also have reduced the efficacy of the compound (Johanson et al., 2004; Kamm et al., 2005).

3. First-in-human trials

3.1 Exposure-response relationship and dose-selection

Single and repeat dose studies are routinely conducted first in healthy volunteers with normal bowel function. The benefit of this approach is the ability to establish preliminary pharmacokinetics and safety profiles in subjects without significant pre-existing conditions. These compounds induce defecatory changes in healthy volunteers, such as increasing bowel movement frequency. However, the doses responsible for these changes in healthy volunteers appear to be higher than the therapeutic dose in chronic constipation patients. GI pharmacodynamic effects in healthy volunteers are dose-dependent and the GI adverse events (i.e., diarrhea) tend to subside after the first dose. In general, there is very limited information on the pharmacokinetic-pharmacodynamic relationship for drugs for this indication. These first-in-man studies are typically followed by pilot dose-ranging safety and efficacy trials in the affected population. Study phases were compressed in the plecanatide program (Shailubhai et al., 2010), which chose to progress to initial repeat-dose studies directly in constipated patients rather than after single-dose studies in normal volunteers. This accelerated approach would seem justified due to the absence of systemic bioavailability and dose accumulation.

In addition to the typical Phase 1 safety studies, gut transit time measurements have been employed to test the prokinetic effects of these compounds in the upper and lower GI tract. These studies have utilized scintigraphic techniques in patients and healthy volunteers (Degen et al., 2001, 2005; Camilleri et al., 2007; Manini et al., 2010; Talley et al., 2006). Endpoints have included colonic transit time (GC24), ascending colon emptying (ACE) $T_{1/2}$, gastric emptying (GE) time and colonic filling at 6 hours (CF6). These endpoints have served as biomarkers for drug effect in the upper and lower GI tract and have guided subsequent indications. Pharmacodynamic endpoints such as scintigraphic transit time are easier to achieve and require fewer subjects than those than those employed in registration trials. This approach minimizes study timeline and cost. It is worth noting that subsequent therapeutic doses for chronic constipation also tend to be lower than the doses needed to demonstrate pharmacodynamic effect in transit studies (Goldberg et al., 2010; Manini et al., 2010).

Dose proportional effects on stool frequency, stool consistency, and other symptoms associated with constipation are ordinarily observed with compounds in both the 5-HT_4 and secretagogue drug classes. With the possible exception of plecanatide, the incidence of diarrhea rises with use of these agents at higher doses. Drugs such as prucalopride, velusetrag, linaclotide, plecanotide, A3309, and RDX-5791 exhibit prolonged pharmacokinetic exposures and/or pharmacodynamic effects and offer the advantage of once daily dosing.

4. Late-stage clinical trials

4.1 Study population

Despite treatment dissatisfaction with OTC medications (Johanson & Kralstein, 2007), there have been no prospective definitions of treatment failure with prior treatment in clinical trials. To date, treatment failure has not been an entry requirement into any late-stage constipation trial. In one of the three pivotal trials that formed the basis of the approval of prucalopride for CIC in Europe in 2009, 87% of subjects with constipation reported dissatisfaction with prior laxative regimens (Tack et al., 2009). Other than this one trial, the concept of treatment refractoriness has not been adequately addressed in registrational trials, which regulatory authorities use to develop label claims. It will be important to make this distinction prospectively if the role of newer medications in the constipation treatment paradigm is to be fully understood. Other study population considerations are outlined in Table 2.

Rome III Criteria (Modified)

- ≤ 3 SBM per week
- One or more of the following symptoms occurring on ≥ 25% of BM for at least 12 weeks during the preceding 12 months
    - Straining during bowel movements
    - Lumpy or hard stools
    - Sensation of incomplete evacuation

Treatment dissatisfaction or failure
Gender
Elderly population (over 65 years of age)
Pelvic floor dyssynergia
Renal or hepatic impairment

Exploratory:
Transit time measurements

Table 2. Key Inclusion/Exclusion Criteria and Considerations in Constipation Trials

It is important to demonstrate safety and efficacy in most patients who are most often affected. In general, CIC is more common in women (Chuong et al., 2007), and not surprisingly, the majority of subjects who have participated in clinical trials have been women. The label claim of prucalopride was restricted to women because the enrollment of low number of male subjects in clinical trials precluded proof of efficacy in men. Although the data are very limited, the effective dose in males may also be higher than females (European Medicines Agency, 2009).

Constipation affects up to 50% of elderly individuals and is especially prevalent in nursing home residents (Camilleri et al., 2009; Chuong et al., 2007; Müller-Lissner et al., 2010). However, pharmacokinetics, the safety and tolerability profile and clinical efficacy in elderly patients may be different than in the younger population. The elderly population is routinely restricted in earlier pharmaceutical development due to safety considerations. The efficacy of prucalopride in the elderly population was demonstrated in a late-stage, multicenter trial of 300 elderly patients (Müller-Lissner et al., 2010). A subsequent safety trial was conducted in frail elderly patients residing in a nursing facility (Camilleri et al., 2009). Dosing should take diminishing renal function into the consideration if the drug is eliminated through the kidney. The effect of age on the pharmacokinetics of prucalopride was studied in an open, parallel-group trial in 12 healthy elderly (age range 65 to 81 years) and 12 young subjects (European Medicines Agency, 2009). Peak plasma concentrations and AUC of prucalopride were 26% to 28% higher in elderly subjects compared with young adults, due to diminishing renal function with age.

Patients participating in late-stage constipation trials should meet established definitions for chronic idiopathic constipation. The Rome II criteria for CIC were published in 1999 (Thompson et al., 1999), and followed by the Rome III criteria in 2006 (Longstreth et al., 2006). Modifications of these criteria have become working standards for inclusion and exclusion in constipation trials. The Rome criteria provide for a history of ≤ 3 SBMs per week and having one or more of the following symptoms for at least 12 weeks during the 12 months preceding the study: (1) straining during ≥ 25% of BMs; (2) lumpy or hard stools during ≥ 25% of BMs; or (3) sensation of incomplete evacuation during ≥ 25% of BMs.

The unmodified Rome III criteria for CIC include the sensation of anorectal obstruction or need for manual maneuvers to facilitate defecation (e.g., digital evacuation, support of the pelvic floor). Approximately 10% of subjects with CIC have functional outlet obstruction associated with pelvic floor dysfunction (Lembo & Camilleri, 2003). Formal radiographic or manometric testing is required to establish the diagnosis. These patients may be less responsive to pharmaceutical approaches than other patients, and are more appropriately treated with biofeedback or surgical methods (Lembo & Camilleri, 2003; Locke et al., 2000). Study protocols have typically tried to exclude patients with a history of dyssynergic defecation or in whom the history and physical examination was felt to indicate the presence of this type of constipation (Johanson et al., 2004; Lembo et al., 2010b).

To confirm the diagnosis of CIC, patients typically undergo a two-week baseline screening period during which time they must report an average of ≤ 3 CSBMs and ≤ 6 SBMs per week for inclusion. The patient responses are generally captured via an electronic diary or interactive voice response system. Use of a laxative, enema, and/or suppository usage for two or more days, or the report of any watery stools (Type 7) or > 1 loose (mushy) stools (Type 6) on the Bristol Stool Form Scale [BSFS] (Lewis & Heaton, 1997) would exclude a patient from participation.

Although constipation is associated with slower colonic transit, only a small portion of patients with CIC have abnormally slow transit times on formal testing (Lembo & Camilleri, 2003). Although transit time measurements may be a useful gauge for the effectiveness of an investigational agent, particularly in the early stages of clinical development, there would appear to be insufficient rationale to qualify patients for late-stage trials based on these transit time measurements.

4.2 Endpoints

Efficacy in constipation trials should signify improvement in constipation-associated symptoms. Endpoints in constipation trials are therefore patient-reported. Regulatory standards for tools to measure symptom-based endpoints in the United States is built on the FDA Guidance for Patient Reported Outcomes, issued in draft form in February 2006 and finalized in December 2009 (US Food and Drug Administration, 2009). Primary efficacy endpoints in late-stage constipation trials typically embody increases in the number of bowel movements (BM) per day, either improvement in spontaneous bowel movements (SBM) or complete spontaneous bowel movements (CSBM) (Table 3). A BM is deemed an SBM if no laxative, enema, or suppository was taken in the preceding 24 hours, and a CSBM if the patient indicated that the SBM is associated with a sensation of complete bowel emptying. Until there is a well-validated patient reported outcome tool the FDA accepts, PRO development will need to be considered in parallel with the clinical development program. In addition, translation and validation of these tools in different languages will also be essential for clinical development plans that expand beyond English speaking populations.

Phase of Development	Instrument	Measurement
First-in-man		
Scintigraphy	Whole gut or colon TT	Geometric center
Stool consistency	BSFS	7-point ordinal scale
Early phase (pilot studies)		
SBM	Daily diary	Average change from baseline
CSBM	Daily diary	Average change from baseline
Late-phase		
Primary endpoint:		
Responder definition CSBM	Daily diary	Categorical variables based on MID
– Achieving of ≥ 3 CSBM/week		
– Increase of ≥ 1 CSBM/week (either co-primary or key secondary endpoint)		
Secondary or exploratory endpoints		
– Stool consistency	BSFS	7-point ordinal scale
– Abdominal pain or discomfort	Severity score	11-point ordinal severity scale
– Straining	Severity score	5-point ordinal severity scale
– Bloating	Severity score	5-point ordinal severity scale
– Use of rescue medications		Change in mean
– PAC-SYM	Composite instrument	Total /domain scores
– PAC-QoL	Composite instrument	Total /domain scores
– Global endpoints		
Constipation severity	Severity score	5-point ordinal severity scale
Global relief of constipation	Numerical rating scale	7-point balanced scale
Treatment satisfaction	Numerical rating scale	5-point ordinal scale
Adequate relief	Binary question	Binary (yes/no)

Table 3. Endpoints in Clinical Trials in Constipation. Abbreviations: *BSFS*, Bristol Stool Form Scale; *TT*, transit time; *MID*, minimally important difference; *CSBM*, complete spontaneous bowel movement; *SBM*, spontaneous bowel movement

The conceptual framework of constipation treatment response embodies symptoms considered important to the patient. These typically include stool consistency, straining, abdominal pain, bloating, and feeling of bowel emptying. Stool consistency is typically measured on the Bristol Stool Form Scale (BSFS). The constipation symptom roster is usually elicited in focus groups of individuals suffering from constipation. Patient responses are then structured into questionnaires using psychometric methods described in the guidance. These symptoms comprise primary and secondary endpoints that form the basis of label claims in the United States.

Earlier stage trials in constipation typically utilize continuous variables, such as mean change in SBM and/or CSBM from baseline across patients groups, for primary efficacy endpoints. These endpoints are easier to power and therefore engender lower sample sizes. Lubiprostone was approved in the US on the basis of trials that employed changes in SBM (Barisch et al., 2010; Johanson et al., 2008). However, the recent guidance makes clear the need for responder definitions in late-stage clinical trials (US Food and Drug Administration, 2009).

Responder definitions should be predicated on subjects achieving minimally important differences (MID) (US Food and Drug Administration, 2009). These differences are derived from factor analyses of clinical data in Phase 2 trials. MIDs are typically determined by comparing symptomatic improvement to global improvement questions. The primary efficacy endpoint in the prucalopride Phase 3 programs utilized the responder definition of ≥ 3 CSBM per week (Camilleri et al., 2008; Quigley et al., 2009; Tack et al., 2009), with the key secondary efficacy endpoint being the proportion of subjects achieving an increase of ≥ 1 CSBM per week. Three CSBM per week, i.e., approximately one BM every other day, represents normalization of bowel function in many individuals (Drossman et al., 1982), and therefore has clinical meaningfulness. The linaclotide Phase 3 program provided for co-primary endpoints that included achieving both ≥ 3 CSBM and improvement of ≥ 1 CSBM/week (Lembo et al., 2010a). The achievement of ≥ 3 CSBM per week is a more stringent and clinically more relevant endpoint than improvement of ≥ 1 CSBM, and efficacy responses on this co-primary endpoint predominantly reflect the subject's response on the first co-primary. It should also be pointed out that CSBM is a more stringent outcome than SBM, and that while endpoints predicated on CSBM may have lower response rates than SBM, the drudging of placebo performance typically results in improved study power, lower sample sizes, and higher chances of trial success.

Drugs have typically achieved responses in the 18% to 29% range on these CSBM-based responder definitions compared with 5% to 15% placebo response in Phase 3 CIC trials. This compares to treatment responses of 30% to 40% using SBM-based definitions, but with higher placebo responses and overall lower levels of statistical significance (Camilleri et al, 2008; Lembo et al, 2010a; Quigley et al, 2009; Tack et al, 2009). The observation that only a quarter of patients normalize bowel function with monotherapy-based trials suggests that the majority of patients will require combination therapy with these agents in the clinic.

Additional efficacy parameters in constipation trials have included the PAC-SYM (Frank et al., 1999), a composite index of constipation-associated symptoms, and PAC-QOL (Marquis et al., 2005), a health-related quality of life instrument, neither of which are recognized by the FDA as acceptable endpoints for clinical trials in the United States. Use of rescue medications and time to first bowel movement have also served as secondary or exploratory endpoints in selected trials. Sponsors have typically included global endpoints such as constipation severity and adequate relief as secondary or exploratory endpoints (Lembo et al., 2010a), and the FDA supports use of these outcomes other than for primary efficacy endpoints (US Food and Drug Administration, 2009).

4.3 Drug safety

Safety concerns are tantamount in drug development for constipation, which is viewed by both clinicians and regulators a non-lifethreatening condition rather than a disease. The tolerance for safety concerns in the treatment of constipation is understandably low. Safety exposure databases should be expected at a minimum to follow ICH Guidelines for chronic disease and include 300-600 six-month exposures and 100 twelve-month exposures (US Food and Drug Administration, 1995). Higher standards may be set by regulatory agencies in the future, and the requirement for risk management programs could be imposed on drugs seeking approval in the US (US Food and Drug Administration, 2005). Pharmacovigilence post-approval has become standard industry practice. When safety is a concern, it is important that drug development identify a minimal effective dose and provide guidance to clinicians on how dosing should be escalated from that point forward. The burden of safety is likely to be reduced for drugs that are locally active compared with those that are systemically available, meaning lower requirements for pre-approval exposures and lower post-approval safety commitments. The GI tract is ideally suited for local or topical exposure by oral or rectal routes of administration.

Potential for QT interval prolongation and drug-drug interactions that potentiate this effect must be identified early in the development program. QT interval prolongation led to the market withdrawal of cisapride in 2000 (Masaoka & Tack, 2009). Tegaserod was associated with a higher incidence of cardiac ischemic events and withdrawn from the market in 2007 (Pasricha, 2007). This concern has shadowed development with all subsequent 5-HT_4 agonists, although current data suggest that QT prolongation and cardiac ischemia may have been due to off-target effects on other receptors or 5-HT receptor subclasses (Chan et al., 2009; DeMaeyer et al., 2008; Serebruany et al., 2010; Tonini et al., 1999). To date, no such events have been observed with prucalopride or any of the current 5-HT_4 development programs.

4.4 Biomarkers

A biomarker is a measureable physical, functional, or biochemical surrogate for a physiological or disease process that has diagnostic and/or prognostic utility (US Food and Drug Administration, 2010a). For many diseases, there is no good way to document the course of a disease or the response to treatment. A biomarker may represent the features of a biologic processes or a response to a therapeutic intervention and reduce the expense and duration of clinical trials. Changes in biomarkers following treatment may reduce uncertainty in drug development by predicting drug performance, identifying safety problems, or revealing pharmacological activity or other benefit from treatment. The European Medicines Agency has also issued guidance for biomarker development in the European Union (European Medicines Agency, 2008).

Radio-opaque markers have been used to assess colonic transit, but recent studies have demonstrated scintigraphic imaging to be a more precise tool for drug development in constipation (Camilleri, 2010; Rao S.S. et al., 2011). Scintigraphic transit time fulfills all regulatory criteria for a disease biomarker: known performance characteristics, reproducible and accurate data over a range of conditions, and evidence of linkage to biological processes and clinical endpoints. Changes in colonic transit by scintigraphic technique have generally predicted the responses to treatment across a variety of compounds (Camilleri, 2010). This may prove to be a biomarker in new drug applications in colonic motility disorders. As noted previously, these transit time measurements define transit time abnormalities in only a minority of patients and are therefore of no specific utility towards defining subjects who enter late-stage clinical trials (Lembo & Camilleri, 2003). Stool frequency correlates poorly with colonic transit, but there appears to be good correlation between gut transit and stool consistency (O'Donnell, Virgie & Heaton, 1990). These markers are generally well accepted and are useful for predicting dose range in subsequent efficacy studies.

5. Clinical trials of approved drugs or drugs in development

5.1 5-HT_4 receptor agonists

5.1.1 Prucalopride

Prucalopride (Resolor®) is a benzofuran carboxamide that is structurally distinct from cisapride and tegaserod. Prucalopride exhibits a more than 2-log scale greater selectivity for 5-HT_4 compared with other receptors (DeMaeyer et al., 2008). This selectivity offers promise for greater efficacy and safety. The 2 mg once daily dose was approved in Europe in 2009 for the treatment of chronic constipation in women who fail to respond to laxatives. Due to the pharmacokinetic considerations described above, it is recommended that the drug be initiated at 1 mg in elderly patients and increased to 2 mg as needed (European Medicines Agency, 2009).

In pharmacodynamic studies, prucalopride dose-dependently enhanced colonic transit both in healthy controls and in patients with chronic constipation. In patients with chronic constipation, prucalopride 2 mg and 4 mg were significantly more effective than placebo in decreasing GI and colonic transit time. This was also reflected in increased stool frequency and looser stool consistency (Bouras et al., 1999, 2001; Sloots et al., 2002). Response in patients with constipation was dose-dependent and effective dosage was generally achieved with 2 mg once daily, although some studies reported significant beneficial effects on 1 mg (Emmanuel et al., 2002; Sloots et al., 2002).

A total of 2717 patients with chronic constipation were treated in placebo-controlled, double-blind, Phase 2 and Phase 3 trials (Miner et al., 1999; Emmanuel et al., 2002; Coremans et al., 2003; Camilleri et al., 2008; Quigley et al., 2009; Tack et al., 2009; Müeller-Lissner et al., 2009). Doses of prucalopride ranged from 0.5 to 4 mg per day. Two of these trials recruited patients who were either resistant to, or dissatisfied with laxatives (Coremans et al., 2003, Tack et al., 2009), one of these being pivotal (Tack et al., 2009), and one trial involved patients aged over 65 years (Müeller-Lissner et al., 2009).

In the Phase 3 program that served as the basis of approval of prucalopride in Europe, three identically designed, multicenter, pivotal trials were conducted (Camilleri et al., 2008; Quigley et al., 2009; Tack et al., 2009). More than 85% of the subjects in these trials were women. Patients were included based on the criteria of two or fewer SBMs per week in the previous 6 months and very hard or hard stools and/or a sensation of incomplete evacuation and/or straining during defecation for at least a quarter of the stools. The primary parameter was the proportion (%) of patients with an average of 3 or more spontaneous, complete bowel movements per week (responders, ≥ 3 CSBM/week). The main secondary endpoint was the proportion of patients with an average increase of ≥ 1 CSBM per week from run-in. The key time-point was assessed at Week 12. Treatment with prucalopride 2 mg and 4 mg once daily resulted in an average of three spontaneous, complete bowel movements (CSBM) per week in 19.5% to 28.5% of subjects treated with prucalopride vs. 9.6% to 13.6% receiving placebo. Significant changes were also seen in the main secondary endpoint.

Clinically relevant improvement in constipation-associated symptoms and quality of life were observed using the PAC-SYM and PAC-QOL questionnaires in these pivotal trials. Nearly 2600 patients were treated with prucalopride in open, long-term studies. 1490 of these subjects received treatment for at least 6 months and 869 received at least 1 year of treatment. The effects of the 2 mg and 4 mg doses of prucalopride were similar, and both were determined to be safe and well tolerated.

Only one cardiovascular event was reported, an episode of supraventricular tachycardia, and extensive cardiovascular safety assessments demonstrated no signals of arrhythmogenic potential (Camilleri et al., 2009). The incidence of serious adverse events was similar to placebo. Headache, nausea, and diarrhea were reported more often in subjects receiving prucalopride, but these adverse events were mainly driven by the occurrence on Day 1 of treatment. It was postulated that this represented a transient effect of 5-HT_4 agonists that penetrate the CNS. However, the relationship between these adverse events and the degree of CNS penetration is inconsistent across this class of compounds.

Data from a series of thorough QT studies appear to show that the influence, if any, of prucalopride on QT interval and other ECG variables is negligible. The number of cardiovascular ischemic-related events was low and comparable between prucalopride groups and placebo (0.1%). Clinical trials with prucalopride were temporarily suspended in 1999 following positive carcinogenicity studies in rodents; however, these findings were deemed to be rodent-specific and were not thought on regulatory review to apply to humans (European Medicines Agency, 2009).

5.1.2 Velusetrag

Velusetrag (TD-5108) is a high-affinity and selective 5-HT_4 receptor agonist with high intrinsic activity at the human 5-HT_4 receptor. Unlike tegaserod, velusetrag has no appreciable affinity for 5-HT_{1D}, 5-HT_{2A}, or 5-HT_{2B} receptors (Beattie et al., 2004; Smith et al., 2007). In contrast to cisapride, velusetrag has no significant affinity for the human ether-a-go-go-related gene potassium channel (Smith et al., 2008). In animal models, velusetrag demonstrated gastrointestinal activity in the digestive tract. To date, no significant effects of velusetrag on blood pressure, heart rate or electrocardiogram have been noted in animals or humans at clinically relevant doses, nor does velusetrag have any contractile activity in porcine- or canine-isolated coronary arteries (Beattie et al. 2007).

A dose-response transit study showed that velusetrag administration was associated with acceleration of colonic and orocecal transit after single dose administration to healthy subjects with substantive and significant effects on gastric and colonic transit were observed with multiple dosing (Manini et al., 2010). In an evaluation of patients with chronic constipation and matched healthy control subjects, velusetrag pharmacokinetics and effects on laxation and bowel function were similar in chronic constipation and health. Bioavailability of velusetrag from a single, orally administrated dose was good, and the elimination half-life in both populations was consistent with once daily administration (Goldberg, Wong, & Ganju 2007; Wong S.L. et al., 2007).

A Phase 2, double-blind, placebo-controlled, randomized, parallel-group, multicenter trial included 401 subjects with chronic idiopathic constipation (< 3 SBM per week) randomized to velusetrag 15 mg, 30 mg, 50 mg or placebo po QD for 4 weeks (Goldberg et al, 2010). The study population was 92% female. Patients receiving velusetrag achieved statistically significant and clinically meaningful increases in SBM and CSBM relative to placebo at all doses. There were no differences in changes in SBM and CSBM rates between doses. Median times with first SBM were 21, 25 and 18 hours, respectively, compared to 47 hours for placebo ($p < 0.0001$ for all treatments). Use of velusetrag was significantly associated with a relief of straining and bloating, a reduced need for a rescue laxative, and normalization of stool consistency.

The most common adverse events in patients were those frequently associated with 5-HT_4 agents such as prucalopride and included diarrhea, headache, and nausea. These adverse events were dose-related, occurred during the initial days of dosing, and were of mild to moderate intensity. A total of 19 patients discontinued because of adverse events, with the majority occurring in the 50 mg velusetrag group. No clinically relevant changes in hematology, biochemistry, urinalysis, vital signs and ECG parameters were observed in any group.

5.1.3 Naronapride

Naronapride (ATI-7505) is a 5-HT_4 receptor agonist belonging to the benzamide series of similar compounds (Camilleri et al, 2007). The design of naronapride was based on the prototypical benzamide agent, cisapride. Unlike cisapride, naronapride was designed to be devoid of other 5-HT receptor activities and to have negligible inhibitory activity at the hERG channel, with an affinity ratio between I_{Kr} and 5-HT_4 receptors of at least 1000- fold. In addition, the compound was to have low potential for drug–drug interactions. Unlike prucalopride and velusetrag, naronapride does not exhibit CNS penetration, which may lead to a lower incidence of side effects (Aryx Corporation, 2008). However, other 5-HT_4 agonist with limited CNS penetration (i.e., tegaserod) did show comparable rate of adverse events to prucalopride and velusetrag.

A randomized, parallel-group, double-blind, placebo-controlled study evaluated effects of 9-day treatment with naronapride (3, 10 or 20 mg TID) on scintigraphic GI and colonic transit in healthy volunteers (12 per group) (Camilleri et al., 2007). Primary endpoints were gastric-emptying (GE) $T_{1/2}$, colonic geometric centre (GC) at 24 h and ascending colon (AC) emptying $T_{1/2}$. Naronapride increased colonic transit with greatest effect vs. placebo observed at 10 mg TID. The effect on transit was associated with looser stool consistency.

A randomized, multinational, multicenter, double-blind, placebo-controlled, dose-ranging trial was performed in patients with CIC (Palme et al., 2010). Patients were randomized to naronapride 20 mg, 40 mg, 80 mg or 120 mg or placebo BID orally for four weeks. Although

400 subjects were planned in the original study design, the study was terminated early due to business reasons, and only 214 patients were randomized. The primary outcome was total number of SBMs during Week 1 compared with placebo. Treatment response, a secondary endpoint, was defined as the proportion of subjects achieving ≥ 3 CSBM/wk or ≥ 3 SBMs/wk on each of the four weeks in the absence of rescue medications. Despite the reduction from the intended original sample size, all doses of naronapride still met the primary endpoint, and median time to first SBM was reduced in all active treatment groups. SBM response was achieved by 51.2% of subjects treated with naronapride 80 mg vs. 24.4% receiving placebo, while CSBM response was achieved by 26.8% of these subjects vs. 4.9% receiving placebo. Adverse event frequency, including headache, diarrhea, nausea and vomiting, was similar to placebo in all ATI-7505 dose groups except the 120 mg BID group, where abdominal pain and headache were more frequently reported.

5.2 Colonic secretagogues

5.2.1 Lubiprostone

Lubiprostone is a poorly absorbed lipophylic prostanoid component that is thought to stimulate colonic water and electrolyte secretion through the activation of type-2 chloride channels on enterocytes from the luminal side (Lacy & Levy, 2007). There is also evidence that the Cl secretion induced by lubiprostone may be mediated by CFTR channels (Bijvelds et al., 2009). Lubiprostone dose-dependently enhances colonic transit, and this was hypothesized to be an indirect consequence of increased colonic water content (Camilleri et al., 2006).

In two Phase 3 studies of 4 weeks duration, lubiprostone 24 mg BID significantly enhanced SBM frequency (5.69 and 5.89 spontaneous bowel movements per week with lubiprostone vs. 3.46 and 3.99 with placebo, $p < 0.0001$) and relieved other constipation-related symptoms compared with placebo (Barish et al., 2010; Johanson et al., 2008). The incidence of nausea in patients receiving the approved dose of lubiprostone for chronic idiopathic constipation was approximately 29% in clinical trials, and resulted in 9% of patients discontinuing in these studies (Lacy & Chey, 2009; Sucampo Pharmaceuticals, 2009). The prevalence of nausea is increased with higher dose and could be mediated by an adverse prostaglandin-like effect on gastric motility (Lacy & Levy, 2007). Although the systemic availability of lubiprostone is reportedly low (Lacy & Levy, 2007), this side effect could potentially reflect systemic absorption post oral administration.

Lubiprostone was approved by the US FDA in 2006 for the treatment of chronic idiopathic constipation (24 mg BID) and for the treatment of female IBS patients with constipation (8 mg BID) (Drossman et al, 2009) in 2008 but, apart from Switzerland, has not been approved in Europe at this time.

5.2.2 Linaclotide

Linaclotide is a 14-amino acid peptide analog of E. coli ST_a enterotoxin that acts as an agonist at guanylate cyclase-C (GCC) receptor to induce cyclic GMP production and intestinal chloride and fluid secretion (Bharucha, Scott & Waldman, 2010). The drug is non-absorbed and exerts local effects on the enterocyte at the level of the gut lumen. In a mechanistic study, linaclotide enhanced colonic transit in IBS with constipation (Andresen et al., 2007). It dose-dependently increased SBM and CSBM frequency, loosened stool consistency, and improved other symptoms of constipation over four weeks (Lembo et al., 2010b).

Favorable outcomes were recently achieved in two large Phase 3 studies, each involving more than 600 subjects, and 12 weeks of treatment. Trial design considered the Food and Drug Administration's recent recommendations to transition from global (e.g., overall relief) to symptom-based primary endpoints (US Food and Drug Administration, 2010b). Subjects were randomized to placebo and 133 or 266 mg of linaclotide (Lembo et al, 2010a). The primary endpoint was based on a responder analysis of subjects achieving both ≥ 3 CSBM and an increase of ≥1 CSBM per week. In both trials, significantly higher percentages of patients met the primary endpoint with linaclotide 133 mg (respectively 16% and 21.2%) and 266 mg (respectively 21.4% and 19.3%) compared with placebo (respectively 6% and 3.3%, all p-values < 0.001). The onset of efficacy occurred in the first week and was maintained for 12 weeks. Symptoms of abdominal discomfort, bloating and straining were also significantly improved. There was also improvement in health-related quality of life, and constipation severity. Linaclotide is also under evaluation for IBS with constipation (Johnston et al, 2010), and an application for marketing approval of linaclotide in the US and Europe for both indications is expected in the near future.

5.2.3 Plecanatide

Plecanatide (SP-304) is an oral peptide analogue of uroguanylin, a natriuretic hormone that regulates ion and fluid transport in the GI tract. T84 cell assays have demonstrated that plecanatide has an 8-fold higher binding affinity to GC-C receptors than uroguanylin. In a double-blind, placebo-controlled, randomized, single ascending dose study conducted in healthy volunteers, plecanatide appeared to demonstrate an increase in post-dose stool consistency score versus placebo (Shailubhai et al., 2008). The drug was well-tolerated at all doses with no systemic exposure. A subsequent Phase 2a trial in constipated subjects studied doses between 0.3 and 9 mg once daily for 14 days (Shailubhai et al., 2010). Dose proportionate reduction in time to first BM, SBM, CSBM, and stool consistency, and improvement of straining were observed up to 1.0 mg, subsequent to which no additional effects were noted. There was no detectable absorption of plecanatide at any dose, and minimal adverse events were observed. There were no reports of diarrhea in any dose groups, although the effects of plecanatide on SBM frequency and stool consistency were less pronounced than in earlier linaclotide trials.

5.2.4 A3309

A3309 is a potent and selective inhibitor of the ileal bile acid transporter (IBAT) with minimal systemic exposure. It dose-dependently inhibits the reabsorption of bile acids (BA). This results in an increased concentration of bile acids in the colon, which, in turn, increase fluid secretion and colonic motility.

In a randomized, double-blind, dose-escalating study, 30 patients were administered A3309 (0.1, 0.3, 1, 3 or 10 mg once daily) or placebo for 14 days (Simrén et al., 2011). Colonic transit was measured using radio-opaque markers and fluoroscopy at baseline and at Day 14. Bowel movements (BMs), stool consistency (Bristol Stool Form Scale) and GI symptoms were recorded daily. Hepatic BA synthesis was estimated by measurement of 7α-hydroxy-4-cholesten-3-one (C4) in peripheral blood. Dose-dependent inhibition of bile acid desorption and acceleration of colonic transit time and SBMs were noted.

In a follow-up trial, 36 female patients were randomized to placebo, 15 mg A3309, or 20 mg A3309 administered orally once daily for 14 consecutive days (Wong B.S. et al., 2011). Whole gastrointestinal and colonic transit, stool consistency, constipation symptoms, serum 7αC4, and fasting serum total and LDL cholesterol (surrogates of inhibition of BA absorption) were measured. Colonic transit at 48h was significantly accelerated with both A3309 dosages. Significantly looser stool consistency, lower constipation severity and straining, and improved ease of stool passage were noted with both A3309 dosages. A3309 treatment significantly and reversibly increased fasting 7αC4. The most common side effect was lower abdominal pain or cramping.

Positive results from a larger, proof-of-concept trial have recently been published (Chey et al., 2011a). 190 patients with severe constipation were treated with 5 mg, 10 mg, or 15 mg A3309 or placebo for 8 weeks. Subjects were mainly female (90%) and averaged 0.4 CSBMs per week at baseline. The primary efficacy endpoint, change from baseline in spontaneous bowel movements (SBMs), showed a dose-dependent increase and highly significant results were obtained for the two highest dose levels. In addition, the secondary endpoints of effects on SBM and CSBM frequencies were also dose dependent and statistically significant. Bloating and straining, important constipation symptoms, also decreased significantly during A3309 treatment. The effect of A3309 was rapid and a significantly higher proportion of the A3309-treated patients had a CSBM within 24 hours of the first administration. The beneficial effects were maintained over the eight-week trial period.

Abdominal pain and diarrhea once again appeared to be the most common side effects with A3309 treatment. These events were observed in 10%, 11%, and 25% and 8%, 11%, and 17%, respectively, in the A3309 5 mg, 10 mg, and 15 mg dose groups, compared with only 0% and 4% in placebo-treated subjects. A similar adverse event profile was recently noted with use of chenodeoxycholic acid in healthy volunteers and female subjects with constipation-predominant IBS (Odynsi-Shiyanbade et al., 2010; Rao A.S. et al., 2010). These observations leave the tolerability of choleretic agent an open-ended question at this time. Increased C4 and reduced LDL cholesterol suggested increased BA synthesis due to inhibition of ileal BA transport. As previously discussed, the long-term effects of this therapeutic approach on fat-soluble vitamin absorption remains to be established.

5.3 Na-H exchange inhibitors

5.3.1 RDX-5791

RDX5791 is a unique, minimally systemic, small molecule NHE3 inhibitor in clinical development for the treatment of CIC. Unlike secretagogues that induce active Cl secretion, RDX5791 inhibits the intestinal Na-H antiport protein (NHE3) that plays a key role in the uptake of sodium and thus water from the intestinal lumen. The most attractive feature of the drug's mechanism is the fact the NHE3 transporter accounts for the principal mechanism of Na and water absorption in humans from duodenum to left colon. Unlike linaclotide, the actions of which may be restricted to the duodenum, RDX5791 may exert its effects along the GI tract. This would theoretically allow for more gradual hydration of stool, and less of a tendency for diarrhea as the dose is increased. The effects of RDX5791 on stool consistency and transit time have been demonstrated in animal models (Spencer et al., 2011). RDX5791 has been demonstrated to be anti-nociceptive in an animal model of visceral hypersensitivity (Eutamene et al., 2011). Pharmacokinetic trials have been completed, and proof-of-concept studies are currently underway in patients with IBS-c.

6. Related indications

6.1 Constipation-predominant irritable bowel syndrome

Drugs that are effective in CIC also appear to be effective in patients with irritable bowel syndrome with constipation (IBS-c). The dual effect on CIC and IBS-c appears to apply to most prokinetic agents and secretagogues. The distinction between CIC and IBS-c patients may be difficult in practice, and it is likely many patients are cross-included in their respective clinical trials. Patients typically qualify for IBS-c trials by fulfilling Rome Criteria for IBS-c and demonstrating of minimal level of abdominal pain on pre-randomization screening diaries, at least 3 out of a possible 10 on a numerical rating scale (Chey et al., 2011b). This practice was recently codified in the FDA IBS draft guidance (U.S. Food and Drug Administration, 2010b). However, while there have been minimum pain requirements to enter IBS-c trials, there have been no maximums that would exclude patients from CIC trials. In fact, it is recognized that a number of patients enter CIC trials reporting baseline pain that exceeds the IBS-c minimum (Lembo et al., 2010b). A retrospective analysis of Phase 3 CIC data demonstrated that CIC patients with a pain score ≥ 3 (on a scale of 10) were as likely to respond to linaclotide as the overall study population (Lembo et al, 2011). Interestingly, patients entering a recent multicenter IBS-c trial with linaclotide demonstrated more severe constipation than those entering CIC trials with the same compound (Johnston et al., 2010).

The mechanism of pain relief in IBS-c most likely relates to decompression of colonic distention, although reduction of visceral hypersensitivity has been suggested using animal models (Eutamene et al., 2009). The mechanism of this anti-nociceptive effect is uncertain, since the phenomenon also appears to apply broadly across a variety of promotility agents that could have utility in CIC and IBS-c (Eutamene et al., 2011, Greenwood-van Meerveld et al., 2006). It has been suggested that stimulation of intracellular c-GMP is responsible for the pain reductions with linaclotide use (Eutamene et al., 2009). However, the mechanism of this effect remains uncertain, since linaclotide is non-absorbed and appears to be released and degraded principally in the duodenum (Kessler et al., 2008), while has been presumed that IBS pain originates in the lower GI tract.

6.2 Opioid-induced constipation

A number of peripherally acting μ-opiate antagonists are currently being investigated for the treatment of opioid-induced constipation (OIC). These drugs are designed not to penetrate or cross the blood brain barrier or adversely impact the efficacy of concomitant analgesic therapy. Methylnaltrexone bromide (Relistor®) has been approved for the treatment of opiate-induced constipation in patients with advanced illness (Thomas et al., 2008). The drug is administered subcutaneously and appears to have onset of effect within four hours. Oral bioavailability has been a challenge, although a new formulation has recently entered Phase 3 trials.

Alvimopan is an orally administered peripherally-acting μ-opioid antagonist approved for the treatment of postoperative ileus (Delaney et al., 2008). In one controlled study in 522 patients on opioids for chronic non-cancer pain, alvimopan in doses of 0.5 mg BID to 2 mg BID was superior to placebo in inducing spontaneous bowel movements and reducing constipation-associated symptoms without antagonism of opioid analgesia (Jansen J.P. et al., 2011; Paulson et al., 2005; Webster et al., 2008), although one of the two pivotal trial failed to meet statistical significance (Irving et al., 2011). This could have resulted from loss of statistical power due to use of SBM rather than CSBM as a primary endpoint, and a placebo response exceeding 50%. Development of alvimopan for OIC was discontinued in 2008 because of a numeric imbalance in myocardial infarction, neoplasm, and bone fracture adverse events that appeared in a long-term safety study.

Several other peripherally-acting μ-opioid antagonists are currently in development for OIC, including TD-1211, NKTR-118, and ALKS-37. One of the challenges will be the development of combination drugs that permit co-administration of opioid with opioid antagonists as a means to prevent constipation from occurring. It is worth noting that opioid antagonists are not expected to cause an increase in the frequency of bowel movements in healthy volunteers or patients with constipation associated with other causes rather than opioid. In contrast, prokinetic agents are likely to improve constipation associated with opioid usage. Lubiprostone and prucalopride are also being studies for the treatment of opioid-induced constipation.

7. Conclusions

Prokinetic agents and secretagogues in development will most likely assume a position on formularies with other constipation therapies, including prucalopride and lubiprostone, and OTC agents. Based on current data, it is unlikely that one agent or class of compounds will suffice for most patients. The challenge will be to integrate different mechanisms into treatment algorithms that optimize safety, cost-effectiveness and therapeutic response. This information will be established in future therapeutic trials.

8. References

Abourmarzouk O.M., Agrawal T., Antakla R., Shariff U., Nelson R.L. (2011). Cisapride for intestinal constipation. Cochrane Database Syst Rev 19: CD007780

Al-Judaibi B., Chande N., Gregor J. (2010). Safety and efficacy of tegaserod therapy in patients with irritable bowel syndrome or chronic constipation. Can J Clin Pharmacol 17:e194–200

Anderson J.L., May H.T., Bair T.L., et al. (2009). Lack of association of tegaserod with adverse cardiovascular outcomes in a matched case-control study. J Cardiovascular Pharmacol Ther 14: 170-175

Andresen V., Camilleri M., Busciglio I.A., et al. (2007). Effect of 5 days linaclotide on transit and bowel function in females with constipation-predominant irritable bowel syndrome. Gastroenterology 133:761–8

Aryx Corporation, Annual Report (2008). http://www.annualreports.com/HostedData/AnnualReports/PDF/aryx2008.pdf

Barish C.F., Douglas Drossman D., Johanson, J.F., Ueno R. (2010). Efficacy and Safety of Lubiprostone in Patients with Chronic Constipation. Dig Dis Sci 55:1090–1097

Beattie D.T., Smith J.A., Marquess D., Vickery R.G. et al. (2004). The 5-HT4 receptor agonist, tegaserod, is a potent 5-HT2B receptor antagonist in vitro and in vivo. Br J Pharmacol 143:549–560

Beattie D.T., Zamora F., Armstrong S.R., Pulido-Rios T., Humphrey P.P.A. (2007) Tegaserod, but not TD-5108, has effects in porcine and canine isolated coronary arteries. Br Pharmacol Soc December meeting P063

Bell T.J., Panchal S.J., Miaskowski C., Bolge S.C., Milanova T., Williamson R. (2009) The prevalence, severity, and impact of opioid-induced bowel dysfunction: results of a US and European Patient Survey (PROBE 1). Pain Med. 10: 35-42

Bharucha A., Camilleri M., Haydock S., et al. (2000). Effects of a serotonin 5-HT(4) receptor antagonist SB-207266 on gastrointestinal motor and sensory function in humans. Gut 47:667-74

Bharucha A.E., Scott A., Waldman S.A. (2010) Taking a lesson from microbial diarrheagenesis in the management of chronic constipation. Gastroenterology 138: 813–25

Bijvelds M.J.C, Bot A.G.M., Escher J.C. and De Jonge H.R. (2009). Activation of Intestinal Cl_ Secretion by Lubiprostone Requires the Cystic Fibrosis Transmembrane Conductance Regulator. Gastroenterology 137:976–985

Borman R.A., Tilford N.S., Harmer D.W., et al. (2002). 5 HT 2B receptors play a key role in mediating the excitatory effects of 5 HT in human colon in vitro. British Journal of Pharmacology135: 1144-1151

Bouras E.P., Camilleri M., Burton D.D., McKinzie S. (1999). Selective stimulation of colonic transit by the benzofuran 5HT4 agonist, prucalopride, in healthy humans. Gut 44:682–643

Bouras E.P., Camilleri M., Burton D.D., et al. (2001). Prucalopride accelerates gastrointestinal and colonic transit in patients with constipation without a rectal evacuation disorder. Gastroenterology 120:354-60

Brown R.T., Zuelsdorff M., Fleming M. (2006). Adverse effects and cognitive function among primary care patients taking opioids for chronic nonmalignant pain. J Opioid Manag. 2006 May-Jun;2(3):137-46

Camilleri M., Bharucha A.E., Ueno R., et al. (2006). Effect of a selective chloride channel activator, lubiprostone, on gastrointestinal transit, gastric sensory, and motor functions in healthy volunteers. Am J Physiol Gastrointest Liver Physiol 290:G942–7

Camilleri M., Vazquez-Roque M.I., et al. (2007). Pharmacodynamic effects of a novel prokinetic 5 HT4 agonist, ATI-7505, in humans. Neurogastroenterol Motil 19: 30-38

Camilleri M., Kerstens R., Rykx A., Vandeplassche L. (2008). A placebo-controlled trial of prucalopride for severe chronic constipation. N Engl J Med 358:2344–54

Camilleri M., Beyens G., Kerstens R., et al. (2009). Safety assessment of prucalopride in elderly patients with constipation: a double-blind, placebo-controlled study. Neurogastroenterol Motil 21, 1256–e117

Camilleri M. (2010). Scintigraphic biomarkers for colonic dysmotility. Clin Pharm Ther 87:748-53

Chan K.Y., DeVries R., Leijten F.P., et al. (2009). Functional characterization of contractions to tegaserod in human isolated proximal and distal coronary arteries. Eur J Pharmacol 619: 61-7

Choung R., Locke G.R., Schleck C., et al. (2007). Cumulative incidence of chronic constipation: a population-based study 1988 - 2003. Aliment Pharmacol Ther 26:1521-8

Chey W.D., Camilleri M., Chang L., Rikner L., Graffner H.A. (2011a)Randomized placebo-controlled phase IIb trial of A3309, a bile acid transporter inhibitor, for chronic idiopathic constipation. Am J Gastroenterol. 2011 May 24 [Epub ahead of print]

Chey W.D., Lembo A., MacDougall J.E. et al (2011b). Efficacy and safety of once-daily linaclotide administered orally for 26 Weeks in patients with IBS-C: Results from a randomized, double-blind, placebo-controlled Phase 3 trial, Digestive Disease Week, Chicago, IL, Abstract 837

Coremans G., Kerstens R., De Pauw M., et al. (2003). Prucalopride is effective in patients with severe chronic constipation in whom laxatives fail to provide adequate relief. Digestion 67:82e9

Debongnie J.C, Phillips S.F. (1978) Capacity of the human colon to absorb fluid. Gastroenterology 74:698–703

Degen L., Matzinger D., Merz M., et al. (2001) Tegaserod, a 5 HT 4 receptor partial agonist accelerates gastric emptying and gastrointestinal transit in healthy male subjects. Aliment Pharmacol Ther 15: 1745-51

Degen L., Petrig C., Studer D., et al. (2005) Effect of tegaserod on gut transit in male and female subjects. Neurogastroenterol Motil 17:821-6

Delaney C.P., Wolff B.G., Viscusi E.R., et al. (2007). Alvimopan for postoperative ileus following bowel resection— a pooled analysis of Phase III studies. Ann Surg 245: 355-63

De Maeyer J.H., Lefebvre R.A., Schuurkes J.A. (2008). 5-HT4 receptor agonists: similar but not the same. Neurogastroenterol Motil 20:99–112

Drossman D.A., Sandler R.S., McKee D.C., et al. (1982). Bowel patterns among subjects not seeking health care. Use of a questionnaire to identify a population with bowel dysfunction. Gastroenterology 83:529–534

Drossman D.A., Chey W.D., Johanson J.F., Fass R., Scott C ., Panas R., et al. (2009). Clinical trial: lubiprostone in patients with constipation- associated irritable bowel syndrome - results of two randomized, placebo-controlled studies. Aliment Pharmacol Ther 29:329–41

Emmanuel A.V., Roy A.J., Nicholls T.J., Kamm M.A. (2002) Prucalopride, a systemic enterokinetic, for the treatment of constipation. Aliment Pharmacol Ther 16:1347-56

European Medicines Agency (2008). CHMP. Biomarkers qualification: Guidance to applicants. www.ema.europa.eu/.../en_GB/document_library/Regulatory_and_procedural_guideline/2009/10/WC500004202.pdf

European Medicines Agency (2009). CHMP assessment report for Resolor, EMEA/664892/2009, www.ema.europa.eu/.../document_library/EPAR__Public_assessment_report/human/001012/WC500053997.pdf

Eutamene H., Bradesi S., LaRauche M., et al. (2009). Guanylate cyclase C-mediated antinociceptive effects of linaclotide in rodent models of visceral pain. Neurogastroenterol Mot 22(3):312-e84

Eutamene H., Charmot D., Navre M., Lionel Bueno L. (2011). Visceral antinociceptive effects of RDX5791, a first-in-class minimally systemic NHE3 inhibitor on stress-induced colorectal hypersensitivity to distension in rats. Digestive Disease Week, Chicago, IL, Abstract 259

Frank L., Kleinman L., Farup C., Taylor L., Miner P. (1999). Psychometric validation of a constipation symptom assessment questionnaire. Scand J Gastroenterol. 34:870-7.

Foxx-Orenstein A., Camilleri M., Szarka L.A., et al. (2005) Non selective opioid antagonist does not increase small intestine or colon transit effect of tegaserod in subjects with constipation predominant-IBS. Neurogastroenterol Motil 17 (Suppl 2): A-43

Gershon M.D. (2004). Review article: serotonin receptors and transporters— roles in normal and abnormal gastrointestinal motility. Aliment Pharmacol Ther 20 (Suppl 7): 3-14

Gershon M.D., Tack J. (2007) The serotonin signaling system: from basic understanding to drug development for functional GI disorders. Gastroenterology 132:397–414

Goldberg M.R., Wong S.L., Ganju J., et al (2007). TD-5108, a selective 5-HT4 agonist with high intrinsic activity, shows immediate and sustained prokinetic activity in healthy subjects. Gastroenterology 2007; 132: A60

Goldberg M., Li Y., Johanson J.F., et al. (2010) Clinical trial: the efficacy and tolerability of velusetrag, a selective 5 HT 4 agonist with high intrinsic activity, in chronic idiopathic constipation - a 4 week, randomized, double blinded, placebo-controlled, dose response study. Aliment Pharmacol Ther 32: 1102-1112

Greenwood-van Meerveld B, Venkova K, Hicks G, et al. (2006) Activation of peripheral 5-HT receptors attenuate colonic sensitivity to intraluminal distension. Neurogastroenterol Mot 18: 76-86.

Harris L.A., Crowell M.D. (2007). Drug evaluation: Linaclotide, a new direction in the treatment of irritable bowel syndrome and chronic constipation. Current Opinion in Molecular Therapeutics 9: 403-410

Higgins P., Johanson J. (2004) Epidemiology of constipation in North America: a systematic review. Am J Gastroenterol 99:750-9

Hoffman J.M., Balemba O.B., Johnson A.C., et al. (2010). Mucosal administration of 5-HT4 receptor agonists enhances colonic motility, inhibits colonic hypersensitivity, and activates 5-HT release. Digestive Disease Week, New Orleans, LA, May 2010, Abstract 861

Huang SM and Woodcock J. (2009). Transporters in drug development:advancing on the Critical Path. Nat Rev Drug Discov. 2010 Mar;9(3):175-6

Irving G., Pénzes J., Ramjattan B., et al (2011). A randomized, placebo-controlled phase 3 trial (study SB-767905/013) of alvimopan for opioid-induced bowel dysfunction in patients with non-cancer pain. J Pain. 12:175-84

Jansen J.P., Lorch D., Langan J., et al (2011). A randomized, placebo-controlled phase 3 trial (Study SB-767905/012) of alvimopan for opioid-induced bowel dysfunction in patients with non-cancer pain. J Pain. 12:185-93

Johanson J.F., Wald A., Tougas G. et al. (2004). Effect of tegaserod in chronic constipation: a randomized, double-blind, controlled trial. Clin Gastroenterol Hepatol 2: 796–805

Johanson J., Kralstein J. (2007). Chronic constipation: a surveyof the patient perspective. Aliment Pharmacol Ther 25:599–608

Johanson J.F., Dan Morton, M.D., Geenen J., M.D., Ueno R. (2008). Multicenter, 4-week, double-blind, randomized, placebo-controlled trial of lubiprostone, a locally-acting type-2 chloride channel activator, in patients with chronic constipation. Am J Gastroenterol 2008;103:170–177

Johnston J.M., Kurtz C.B., MacDougall J.E., et al. (2010). Linaclotide improves abdominal pain and bowel habits in a Phase IIb study of patients with irritable bowel syndrome with constipation. Gastroenterology 139:1877–1886

Kalso E., Edwards J.E., Moore R.A., McQuay H.J. (2004). Opioids in chronic non-cancer pain: systematic review of efficacy and safety. Pain 112:372-80

Kamm M.A., Müller-Lissner S., Talley N.J. et al. (2005). Tegaserod for the treatment of chronic constipation: a randomized, double-blind, placebo-controlled multinational study. Am J Gastroenterol 100:362-72

Kessler M.M., Busby R., Wakefield R.W., et al. (2008) Rat intestinal metabolism of linaclotide, a therapeutic agent in clinical development for the treatment of IBS-C and chronic constipation, International Society for the Study of Xenobiotics, San Diego, CA, October 2008, Abstract 292

Lacy B.E., Levy L.C. (2007). Lubiprostone: a chloride channel activator. J Clin Gastroenterol 41:345–51.

Lacy B.E., Chey WD. (2009) Lubiprostone: chronic constipation and irritable bowel syndrome with constipation. Exp Opinion Pharmacother 10: 143–52

Lee A. and Kuo B, (2010). Metoclopramide in the treatment of diabetic gastroparesis. Exp Rev Endocrin Metab 5: 653-662

Lembo A, Camilleri M. (2003). Chronic constipation. N Engl J Med 349:1360-8

Lembo A., Schneier H., Lavins B.L., et al. (2010a) Efficacy and safety of once daily linaclotide administered orally for 12-weeks in patients with chronic constipation: Results from 2 randomized, double-blind, placebo-controlled Phase 3 trials. Gastroenterology 139: S53–4

Lembo A., Kurtz C.B., MacDougall J.E., et al. (2010b). Efficacy of Linaclotide for Patients With Chronic Constipation. Gastroenterology 138; 886-895

Lembo A., Schneier H., Levins B.J., et al. (2011) The effect of linaclotide on measures of abdominal and bowel symptoms in patients with chronic constipation and abdominal pain: pooled results from two Phase 3 trials. Digestive Disease Week, Chicago, IL, Abstract 214

Lewis S.J., Heaton K.W. (1997). Stool form scale as a useful guide to intestinal transit time. Scand J Gastroenterol 32:920–924

Locke G.R., Pemberton J.H., Phillips S.F. (2000). American Gastroenterological Association medical position statement: Guidelines on constipation. Gastroenterology 199: 1761-78

Longstreth G.F., Thompson W.G., Chey W.D., Houghton L.A., Mearin F., Spiller R.C. (2006). Functional bowel disorders. Gastroenterology 130: 1480–91

Loughlin J., Quinn S., Rivero E., et al. (2010) Tegaserod and the Risk of Cardiovascular Ishemic Events: An observational Cohort Study. J Cardiovasc Pharmacol Therap 15, 151-157

Manini M.L., Camilleri M., Goldberg M., et al. (2010). Effects of Velusetrag(TD 5108) on gastrointestinal transit and bowel function in health and pharmacokinetics in health and constipation. Neurogastroenterol Mot 22: 42-9

Marquis P., De La Loge C., Dubois D., McDermott A., Chassany O. (2005). Development and validation of the Patient Assessment of Constipation Quality of Life questionnaire. Scand J Gastroenterol 40: 540–51

Masaoka T. and Tack J. (2009). Gastroparesis: current concepts and management. Gut and Liver 3: 166-173

Metozolv ODT Prescribing Information (2009), Salix Pharmaceuticals, Morrisville, N.C.

Miner P.B., Nichols T., Silvers D.R., et al. (1999). The efficacy and safety of prucalopride in patients with chronic constipation. Gastroenterology 116(Suppl): A1043

Motola G., Mazzeo F., Rinaldi B., Capuano A., Rossi S., Russo F., et al. (2002). Self-prescribed laxative use: a drug-utilization review. AdvTher 19: 203–8

Müller-Lissner S., Rykx A., Kerstens R., vander Plassche L. (2010) Double-blind, placebo-controlled study of prucalopride in elderly patients with chronic constipation. Neurogastroenterol Mot 22: 991-e255

O'Donnell L.J.D., Virjee J., Heaton K.W. (1990) Detection of pseudodiarrhoea by simple clinical assessment of intestinal transit rate. Br Med J 300:439–440

Odynsi-Shiyanbade S.T., Camilleri M., Mc Kinzie C., et al. (2010). Effects of Chenodeoxycholate and a Bile Acid Sequestrant, Colesevelam on Intestinal Transit and Bowel Function. Clin Gastroenterol Hepatol 8:159–165

Palme M., Milner P.G., Ellis D.J., et al. (2010) A novel gastrointestinal prokinetic, ATI-7505, increased spontaneous bowel movements (SBMs) in a phase II, randomized, placebo-controlled study of patients with chronic idiopathic constipation (CIC). Digestive Disease Week, New Orleans, LA, May 2010, Abstract 905

Pasricha P.J. (2007). Desperately seeking serotonin…A commentary on the withdrawal of tegaserod and the state of drug development for functional and motility disorders. Gastroenterology 132: 2287-90

Paulson D.M., Kennedy D.T., Donovick R.A., et al. (2005). Alvimopan: an oral, peripherally acting, mu-opioid receptor antagonist for the treatment of opioid-induced bowel dysfunction - a 21-day treatment randomized clinical trial. J Pain 6:184–92

Prather C.M., Camilleri M., Zinsmeister A.R., et al. (2000). Tegaserod accelerats orocecal transit in patients with constipation-pre-dominant irritable bowel syndrome. Gastroenteroloty 118: 463-468

Quigley E.M.M, VanderPlasshe R., Kerstens R, and Ausma J. (2009). Clinical trial: the efficacy, impact on quality of life, and safety and tolerability of prucalopride in severe chronic constipation-- a 12-week, randomized, double-blind, placebo-controlled study. Aliment Pharmacol Ther 29, 315–328

Ramkumar D., Rao S.S. (2005). Efficacy and safety of traditional medical therapies for chronic constipation: systematic review. Am JGastroenterol 100:936–71

Rao A.S., Wong B.S., Camilleri M.C., et al. (2010). Chenodeoxycholate in Females With Irritable Bowel Syndrome-Constipation: A Pharmacodynamic and Pharmacogenetic Analysis. Gastroenterology139:1549–1558

Rao S.S., Camilleri M., Hasler W.L., et al (2011). Evaluation of gastrointestinal transit in clinical practice: position paper of the American and European Neurogastroenterology and Motility Societies. Neurogastroenterol Mot 23(1):8-2

Serebruany V.L., Mouelhi M.E., Pfannkuche H.J., et al. (2010). Investigations on 5 HT 4 receptor expression and effects of Tegaserod on human platelet aggregration in vitro. Amer J Therapeutics 17: 543-552

Shah N., Chitkara D., Locke G., et al. (2008). Ambulatory care for constipation in the United States, 1993 - 2004. Am J Gastroenterol 103:1746-53

Shailubhai K, Gerson W, Talluto C, et al. (2008) A randomized, doubleblind,placebo-controlled, single-, ascending-, oral-dose safety, tolerability and pharmacokinetic study of SP-304 in healthy adult human male and female volunteers. Digestive Disease Week. San Diego, CA

Shailubhai K., Talluto C., Comiskey S., PhD, et al. (2010). Phase II clinical evaluation of SP-304, a guanylate cyclase-C agonist, for treatment of chronic constipation. Am J Gastroenterol 105 (Supplement 1s) Supp: S487

Simrén M., Bajor A., Gillberg P.G., et al. (2011). Randomised clinical trial: The ileal bile acid transporter inhibitor A3309 vs. placebo in patients with chronic idiopathic constipation--a double-blind study. Aliment Pharmacol Ther. 34:41-50

Sloots C.E., Poen A.C., Kerstens R., et al. (2002). Effects of prucalopride on colonic transit, anorectal function and bowel habits in patients with chronic constipation. Aliment Pharmacol Ther 16:759-67

Smith J.A.M., Beattie D.T., Cuthbert A.W., et al. (2007). TD-5108, a selective, high intrinsic activity 5-HT4 receptor agonist—in vitro profile at human recombinant 5-HT4 receptor splice variant and human isolated colon. Digestive Disease Week, Washington, DC, W1222

Smith J.A.M., Beattie, D.T., Marquess D., et al. (2008). The in vitro pharmacological profile of TD-5108, a selective 5-HT4 receptor agonist with high intrinsic activity. Naunyn-Schmiedeberg's Arch Pharmacol 378:125–137

Spencer A.G., Jeffrey W. Jacobs J.W., Michael R. Leadbetter M.R.et al (2011), Rdx5791, a first-in-class minimally systemic NHE3 inhibitor in clinical development for CIC and IBS-C, increases intestinal sodium leading to enhanced intestinal fluid volume and transit. Digestive Disease Week, Chicago, IL, Abstract 513

Sucampo Pharmaceuticals, Inc. (2009). AMITIZA (Lubiprostone) Prescribing Information.

Talley N.J., Camilleri M., Burton D., et al. (2006). Double-blind, randomized placebo-controlled study to evaluate the effect of tegaserod gastric motor, sensory and myoelectric function in healthy volunteers. Aliment Pharmacol Ther 24:859-867

Tack J., Müller-Lissner S. (2009). Treatment of chronic constipation: current pharmacologic approaches and future directions. Clin Gastroenterol Hepatol 7:502–8

Tack J., van Outryve M.,Beyens G., Kerstens R., L Vandeplassche L. (2009). Prucalopride (Resolor) in the treatment of severe chronic constipation in patients dissatisfied with laxatives. Gut 58:357–365.

Tack J., Müller-Lissner S., Stanghellini V., Boeckxstaens G., Kamm M.A., Simren M., et al. (2011). Diagnosis and treatment of chronic constipation - a European perspective. Neurogastroenterol Motil 23:697-710

Thomas J., Karver S., Cooney G.A., et al. (2008). Methylnaltrexone for opioid-induced constipation in advanced illness. N Engl J Med 358:2332–43

Thompson W.G., Longstreth G.F., Drossman D.A., et al. (1999). Functional bowel disorders and functional abdominal pain. Gut 45(Suppl II):II43–II47

Tonini M., de Ponti F., di Nucci A., Crema F. (1999). Review article: cardiac adverse effects of gastrointestinal prokinetics. Aliment Pharmacol Ther 13:1585–91

Tramonte S., Brand M., Mulrow C., Amato M., O'Keefe M., Ramirez G. (1997). The treatment of chronic constipation in adults:a systematic review. J Gen Intern Med 12:15–24

U.S. Food and Drug Administration, Center for Drug Evaluation and Research (1995). The extent of population exposure to assess clinical safety: for drugs intended for long-term treatment of non-life-threatening conditions, ICH E1A, http://www.fda.gov/downloads/Drugs/ GuidanceComplianceRegulatoryInformation/Guidances/UCM073083.pdf

U.S. Food and Drug Administration, Center for Drug Evaluation and Research (2005). Guidance for industry: Premarketing risk assessment. http://www.fda.gov/downloads/ RegulatoryInformation/Guidances/UCM126958.pdf

U.S. Food and Drug Administration, Center for Drug Evaluation and Research (2009). Guidance for industry: Patient-Reported Outcome Measures: Use in medical product development to support labeling claims. http://www.fda.gov/downloads/Drugs/GuidanceCompliance RegulatoryInformation/Guidances/UCM193282.pdf

U.S. Food and Drug Administration, Center for Drug Evaluation and Research (2010a). Guidance for industry: Qualification process for drug development tools. http://www.fda.gov/downloads/ Drugs/GuidanceComplianceRegulatoryInformation/Guidances/UCM230597.pdf

U.S. Food and Drug Administration, Center for Drug Evaluation and Research (2010b). Guidance for industry: Irritable bowel syndrome— clinical evaluation of products for treatment. http://www.fda.gov/downloads/Drugs/GuidanceComplianceRegulatoryInform ation/Guidances/UCM205269.pdf

Webster L., Jansen J.P., Peppin J., et al. (2008). Alvimopan, a peripherally acting mu-opioid receptor (PAMOR) antagonist for the treatment of opioid-induced bowel dysfunction: results from a randomized, double-blind, placebocontrolled, dose-finding study in subjects taking opioids for chronic non-cancer pain. Pain 15;137:428–40

Wiseman L. and Faulds D. (1994). Cisapride: An updated review of its pharmacology and therapeutic efficacy as a prokinetic agent in gastrointestinal motility disorders. Drugs 47: 116-152

Wong B. S, Camilleri M., McKinzie S., et al. (2011) Effects of A3309, an Ileal Bile Acid Transporter Inhibitor, on Colonic Transit and Symptoms in Patients with Functional Constipation, Digestive Disease Week, Chicago, IL, Abstract 908

Wong S.L., Goldberg M.R., Shaw J. et al. (2007) In healthy subjects, TD-5108, a selective high intrinsic activity 5- HT4 receptor agonist, shows dose proportional pharmacokinetics and exhibits a profile consistent with once-daily dosing. Gastroenterology 132: A374